ESSENTIAL OILS
& AROMATHERAPY
Bible

7in1

Unleash the Power of Nature's Aromas | The Complete
Guide to Natural Essential Oils and Aromatherapy for
Health, Beauty, Relaxation, and Well-Being

LENA FARROW

TABLE OF CONTENTS

INTRODUCTION

In a world that often moves at a relentless pace, where stress and demands can weigh heavily on our shoulders, we find ourselves yearning for moments of solace and tranquility. Our modern lives, though filled with conveniences and advancements, have also distanced us from the natural remedies that have graced the Earth for centuries. The hustle and bustle have led us to seek refuge in the soothing embrace of nature to rediscover the timeless healing powers that lie within essential oils and aromatherapy.

Welcome to *The Essential Oils and Aromatherapy Bible*, where we embark on an enlightening journey into the heart of holistic well-being. Within these pages lies a treasure trove of wisdom, a comprehensive guide to embracing the ancient practices that tap into the innate potential of Mother Nature. This book endeavors to unlock the mysteries and miracles contained within essential oils and aromatherapy, allowing you to harness their boundless potential for health, beauty, relaxation, and overall well-being.

This literary masterpiece endeavors to be your guiding light in navigating the rich, aromatic world of essential oils and the restorative practices of aromatherapy. It aspires to be your compass, helping you traverse the vast landscape of information and make informed choices that align with your desire for a more holistic and harmonious life.

As we journey through these pages, we will delve into the essence of essential oils, understanding their origins, properties, and the diverse ways in which they can enhance our daily lives. We will unravel the secrets of aromatherapy—the art and science of utilizing aromatic plant extracts for improving physical, emotional, and mental well-being. Together, we will explore the potential of aromatherapy in skincare and beauty, in creating tranquil and rejuvenating environments, and in supporting our bodies through natural healing processes.

This compendium is an invitation to rediscover the ancient wisdom that our ancestors revered—a wisdom that has been passed down through generations, nurturing and healing both body and soul.

The essential oils and aromatherapy we delve into aren't just about fragrances and pleasing scents; they are about holistic wellness, connecting with nature, and embracing the purest, most authentic version of ourselves.

In a world where synthetic solutions are often sought, this book advocates for a return to the roots, to the natural remedies that have stood the test of time. It calls upon you to embrace the wisdom that has been bestowed upon us by the bounteous Earth—a wisdom that has evolved and flourished for millennia. Through the gateway of essential oils and aromatherapy, we can experience a profound transformation—a rejuvenation that encompasses not only the physical but also the emotional and spiritual aspects of our being.

So, let us embark on this odyssey together as we uncover the vast array of essential oils and their therapeutic potential, as we learn the art of blending and application, and as we explore the depths of aromatherapy's healing embrace. The journey is poised to be enlightening, transformative, and, above all, deeply gratifying. Open your heart and senses to the wonders that await, for within these pages lies the roadmap to a more harmonious and vibrant life—a life enriched by the essential oils and aromas of nature.

BOOK 1
INTRODUCTION TO ESSENTIAL OILS AND AROMATHERAPY

CHAPTER 1

UNDERSTANDING ESSENTIAL OILS

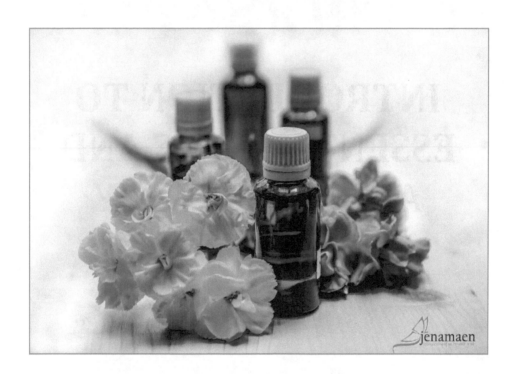

Essential oils are concentrated, volatile plant extracts that capture the natural scent, flavor, and therapeutic properties of the plant source. They have been used for centuries across many cultures for their health, beauty, aromatic and spiritual benefits. This chapter will provide a comprehensive overview of essential oils, how they are produced, their chemical composition, and their mechanisms of action in the body.

What Are Essential Oils?

Essential oils, also referred to as volatile oils, ethereal oils or aetherolea, are hydrophobic liquids extracted from plants through distillation. The term "essential" refers to the fact that these oils capture the quintessential fragrance and therapeutic properties of the plant. Essential oils are found within the leaves, stems, flowers, bark or roots of plants and trees. Through distillation, the volatile aromatic compounds of the plant separate from the water-based compounds to produce a concentrated, hydrophobic oil with the characteristic scent of that plant.

Essential oils are made up of complex mixtures of organic chemicals, primarily terpenes, terpenoids, phenylpropanoids, esters, alcohols, ketones, aldehydes and oxides. These natural aromatic compounds give each essential oil its unique fragrance and therapeutic benefits. For example, the major constituents in lavender essential oil—such as linalool and linalyl acetate—give lavender its sweet floral aroma and calming, relaxing properties. While in peppermint essential oil, menthol is the primary component responsible for its cooling, invigorating, minty scent.

When properly diluted or diffused into the air, essential oils provide pleasing natural fragrances that can uplift mood, help relaxation, and provide other benefits. Essential oils also have topical and internal applications when used appropriately under the guidance of an aromatherapy practitioner.

How Are Essential Oils Made?

Essential oils are extracted from plant materials using a process called distillation. Distillation involves heating plant materials like leaves, flowers, bark, roots or resin to very high temperatures in a still, which separates the aromatic essential oil from the water-based plant compounds.

There are a few main methods of distillation used to extract essential oils:

Steam Distillation

The most common method, steam distillation, passes hot steam through the plant material. The heat causes the oil pockets within the plant to vaporize. As the steam condenses, the water and essential oil separate and the oil floats to the top, where it can be collected. Common oils extracted through steam distillation include lavender, eucalyptus, peppermint and tea tree.

Solvent Extraction

Solvents like hexane or ethanol can also be used to extract essential oils, though this method is being phased out due to the safety hazards of solvent residues. Jasmine, tuberose, carnation, gardenia and jonquil oils are often produced through solvent extraction.

Cold Pressing

Mostly used for citrus essential oils, cold pressing involves mechanically pressing the oil from the rind of citrus fruits. Oils like lemon, sweet orange, grapefruit, mandarin and lime are cold-pressed.

CO2 Extraction

This newer carbon dioxide extraction method puts pressurized CO_2 in a supercritical state that acts as a solvent to extract and isolate essential oils. It is considered a cleaner and safer alternative to solvent extraction. The process is used for delicate flowers like rose and lavender.

Expression

Some essential oils, like lemon oil, are simply expressed by hand squeezing or mechanically pressing the rinds of citrus fruits.

Enfleurage

Labor-intensive enfleurage involves placing fresh flower petals on solid sheets of odorless plant fat or oil and allowing them to infuse, leaving behind pure essential oils slowly. Extraction can take days or weeks. It is mostly used for delicate, expensive flower oils like jasmine, tuberose and rose.

Other methods like maceration, resin tapping and phytonic process are sometimes used for select plant materials. The resulting essential oils are then gently distilled to remove any water and carefully bottled to prevent oxidation. Reputable essential oil companies will declare the botanical origins and extraction methods used to create their oils.

Composition of Essential Oils

Essential oils are made up of a complex array of organic plant chemicals or phytochemicals. While each essential oil has a unique composition, most are composed primarily of terpenes and terpenoids, aromatic phenylpropanoids, and other active organic chemicals like esters, oxides, alcohols, ketones, aldehydes and more. Here is an overview of the major phytochemical constituents in essential oils:

Terpenes and Terpenoids

Terpenes are hydrocarbons produced in the mevalonic acid biological synthesis pathway in plants. They form the basic structure of carotenoids, sterols, latex and essential oils. Terpenes have an isoprene skeleton and can differ in the number of isoprene units they contain. Monoterpenes have two isoprene units, sesquiterpenes have three, and so on. Common terpenes found in essential oils include limonene, pinene, terpinene, sabinene, myrcene, camphene, caryophyllene, humulene, and bisabolol. Terpenoids are oxidized terpenes.

Phenylpropanoids

Derived from the amino acid phenylalanine, phenylpropanoids have a 6-carbon aromatic ring with a 3-carbon propene tail. Common phenylpropanoids in essential oils include eugenol, safrole, cinnamaldehyde, methyl chavicol and estrogen. They have been shown to have antioxidant, anti-inflammatory, anticarcinogenic and immune-stimulating effects in studies.

Esters

Esters are formed by the reaction of alcohols and acids, giving off water as a byproduct. Common esters contributing pleasant fruity and floral notes to essential oils include linalyl acetate, geranyl acetate, eugenyl acetate and bornyl acetate.

Ketones

Ketones contain a carbonyl group linked to two other carbon atoms. They are formed through oxidation and decomposition of carotenoids. Common ketone constituents include jasmone, verbenone, camphor and carvone.

Alcohols

Essential oil alcohols are derived from terpene alcohols. They include geraniol, linalool, citronellol, menthol, borneol, nerol, and farnesol. Alcohols have noted antimicrobial effects.

Aldehydes

Aldehydes contain a formyl group bound to hydrogen and an R group. In essential oils, they are mostly derived from the oxidation of primary alcohols. Prominent aldehydes include citral, citronellal, cinnamaldehyde, and vanillin.

Oxides

Oxides result from exposing an essential oil to oxygen, creating new compounds through oxidation. Common examples are 1,8-cineole, linalool oxide, ascaridole, and bisabolone oxide. Oxides can alter the overall fragrance profile.

The specific proportions of these phytochemical constituents determine the scent, properties, and safety considerations for each essential oil. Analyzing the chemical profile through chromatography allows quality assurance for purity and standardization.

Mechanisms of Action

Essential oils have been shown to exert complex pharmacological and biological effects through a variety of mechanisms of action:

Inhalation Effects

- Olfactory receptors in the nose are triggered, stimulating the limbic system and emotional centers of the brain.
- Lung inhalation allows absorption into the bloodstream for wider bodily effects.

Topical Effects

- Skin absorption allows permeation into the bloodstream for wider effects
- Antimicrobial actions limit infections when applied to the skin
- Anti-inflammatory actions reduce swelling and skin irritation
- Vasodilatory effects improve superficial blood flow

Internal Effects

- Oral ingestion, suppositories or injections allow direct absorption into the bloodstream.
- Interactions with enzymes, hormones, neurotransmitters, cytokines
- Anti-inflammatory, muscle relaxant, diuretic or other effects

Detoxification Support

- Antioxidant activity counteracts free radicals
- Liver enzyme induction aids the body's detoxification process
- Kidney stimulation supports renal elimination
- Lymphatic drainage assisted through massage

The next sections will explore the evidence behind these mechanisms in greater detail, outlining the research on inhalation and topical and internal administration routes.

Methods of Administration

Essential oils can be utilized in several ways: through inhalation, topical application, and oral or internal use. Various factors determine the appropriate application methods for essential oil, including its chemistry, pharmacology, safety data and the desired therapeutic effects. Here is an overview of the major essential oil administration routes:

Inhalation

Inhaling essential oil molecules allows them to rapidly reach receptor sites in the nasal cavity and lungs. Volatile compounds pass easily into the lungs and diffuse into the bloodstream for widespread distribution. Effects are stimulated within seconds to minutes.

- Diffusion: Oils passively dispersed in air via diffuser devices
- Direct Inhalation: Directly breathing in oils from hands, cotton ball, steam tent
- Dry Evaporation: A few drops are allowed to evaporate from an opened bottle

Topical Application

Applying oils to the skin, hair, or nails allows absorption while minimizing potential sensitivity reactions compared to ingestion. Effects manifest within minutes to hours.

- Massage: Oils mixed with carrier oil and massaged into the skin
- Compresses: Oils diluted and applied to hot or cold wet cloth on the skin
- Baths: Dispersed in hot bath water for absorption through the skin
- Hair and Scalp Oils: Applied diluted or undiluted to hair and scalp

Oral Ingestion

Taken by mouth, oils directly enter the digestive tract and bloodstream rapidly. Great care must be taken with internal use due to safety concerns. Effects occur within minutes.

- Oral Use: Dropped into water, under the tongue, in capsule/liquid extracts
- Suppositories: Mixed with carrier oils and introduced rectally
- Vaginal Administration: Very diluted oils are introduced gently into the vagina

The appropriate method depends on the goal, condition, oil chemistry and safety factors. A qualified aromatherapy practitioner can advise on usage based on the individual. Research continues to emerge on safe, effective essential oil application techniques for various situations.

Essential Oil Inhalation

Inhalation is the fastest way to utilize essential oils, as aroma compounds pass quickly into the lungs and diffuse into the bloodstream, reaching the brain and body tissues within seconds to minutes. Breathing in essential oils stimulates smell receptors that signal regions of the limbic system and amygdala in the brain associated with memory, emotion, hormone balance and other involuntary functions. Clinical research has demonstrated meaningful psychological and physiological effects from essential oil inhalation.

Mood Enhancement

Multiple studies reveal inhalation of essential oils can modulate mood, reduce anxiety and stress, alleviate depression symptoms, boost cognition and induce calm or energized states. For example, lemon oil increased alertness, and lavender oil improved relaxation in randomized controlled trials. Brain imaging studies show aromatic compounds communicate with limbic emotional centers, explaining mood-enhancing effects.

Hormone Interactions

Inhalation of essential oils like clary sage, thyme, sage, jasmine and rose has been shown to influence hormone levels, potentially reducing cortisol, estrogen and thyroid hormones. Effects are likely mediated through olfactory stimulation of the hypothalamus and pituitary glands. This provides a mechanism for managing conditions like PMS, menopause and stress.

Immune Stimulation

Inhaled essential oils interact with cytokines, phagocytes and other immune factors to potentially stimulate the immune system. In studies, oils like ylang-ylang, oregano, cinnamon bark, clove bud, rosemary and thyme demonstrated immune-enhancing properties. This makes aromatherapy a useful complementary therapy for immune support.

Congestion Relief

Mentholated essential oils such as peppermint, eucalyptus and camphor have an affinity for bronchial and sinus passages, providing cooling relief and helping respiratory airflow when inhaled or vaporized. This makes them useful for temporary relief of congestion and respiratory discomfort.

Antimicrobial Effects

Certain essential oils exhibit direct antimicrobial effects against pathogenic bacteria, viruses, fungi and molds when vaporized into the air. Oils such as cinnamon, oregano, clove bud, lemon, thyme and tea tree can sanitize air and surfaces. This provides protective properties when diffused into living spaces.

CHAPTER 2

HISTORY AND PRINCIPLES OF AROMATHERAPY

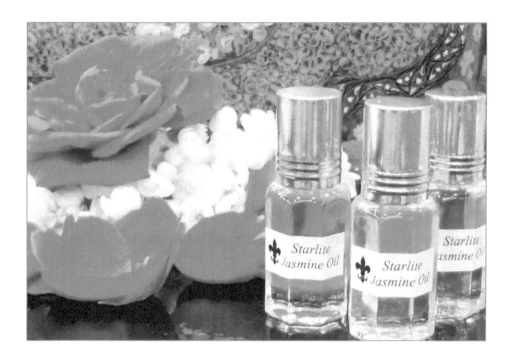

Aromatherapy is the therapeutic use of aromatic plant oils, including essential oils, for holistic healing and wellbeing. The history of aromatherapy is ancient, intricate and rich, spanning numerous cultures and millennia. This chapter explores the origins and evolution of aromatherapy from ancient civilizations to modern times. We will trace how aromatherapy principles developed across the ages and outline the mechanisms by which aromatherapy promotes balance on physiological, psychological, and spiritual levels.

Origins in Ancient Civilizations

The roots of aromatherapy stretch back over 6,000 years to traditional healing systems of ancient Egypt, China, India, Greece, and Rome that incorporated aromatic plant oils. Hieroglyphs show Egyptians developed complex distillation methods to extract essential oils like cinnamon, cedarwood and frankincense for medical and embalming uses. Chinese medicine utilized aromatics like camphor and sandalwood. India's Ayurveda elaborately prescribed aromatherapy massage. Greek and Roman texts documented numerous distillation techniques and health applications of botanical oils. Across these cultures, aromatics served therapeutic, spiritual and ceremonial purposes.

The Middle Ages into Modern Times

References to aromatherapy appeared through the Middle Ages in alchemy texts and folk medicine traditions that drew upon ancient Greek and Arabic knowledge. However, the art of distillation was often shrouded in secrecy. The modern resurgence of aromatherapy began in the early 20th century. French chemist Rene-Maurice Gattefosse coined the term "aromatherapie" after burning his hand and plunging it into lavender oil, amazed at how rapidly it healed. His 1937 seminal text "Gattefosse's Aromatherapy" on essential oils popularized aromatherapy in Europe. French medical doctor Jean Valnet furthered research and used essential oils to treat injured soldiers during World War II.

As scientific studies expanded in the 1950s-1970s, Marguerite Maury opened the first aromatherapy clinic in London in 1964. Austrian biochemist Marguerite Maury systemized modern aromatherapy practices. Robert B. Tisserand published influential essential oil safety guidelines. Nurses like Jeanette Jacknin, Jane Buckle and Roberta Wilson introduced aromatherapy into modern hospital settings. In the 1980s-90s, aromatherapy gained major popularity as a holistic healing modality that continues today.

Principles of Aromatherapy

Aromatherapy utilizes aromatic essential oils derived from carefully extracted and distilled botanical sources. It aims to improve physical, emotional and spiritual wellbeing through therapeutic applications of these plant essences. Key principles of aromatherapy include:

Holistic Focus

Aromatherapy addresses the whole person, including mind, body and spirit. It seeks to bring balance and nourishment physically, mentally, emotionally and energetically.

Nature Synergy

Essential oils synergistically work with innate self-healing abilities to foster vitality by supporting body systems and natural defenses.

Non-Invasive

Aromatherapy provides a non-invasive, pleasurable way to restore health without aggressive medications or treatments that disturb natural functions.

Patient-Centered

Customized protocols are tailored to each individual's presenting needs, sensitivities, preferences and environment for personalized therapeutic benefit.

Whole Plant Potency

Essential oils offer a concentrated form of a plant's healing messages, allowing efficient delivery of its living energy in a potent, bioavailable form.

Empowerment

Aromatherapy encourages self-care through simple, safe methods that restore health while connecting users to the sensory joys and plant wisdom of nature.

Scope of Practice

Aromatherapists work within a scope of practice that allows the recommendation of essential oils while referring to licensed healthcare providers for diagnosing or treating disease.

Aromatherapy Mechanisms of Action

Essential oils promote healing through several mechanisms of action working in synergy. These include physiological, psychological, olfactory and energetic/spiritual effects:

Physiological Effects

Essential oil constituents interact on a cellular level to optimize physical functioning and promote self-regulating homeostasis. Documented effects include:

- Anti-inflammatory, antioxidant, antifungal, antimicrobial, antiviral
- Hormone balancing, menstrual regulating, decongestant
- Analgesic pain relief, antispasmodic muscle relaxant
- Digestive stimulant or soothing, circulatory stimulant effects

Psychological Effects

Inhaled essential oil molecules communicate with the limbic region of the brain linked to memory, mood and behavior. This gives oils psychoactive properties that can:

- Improve depression, anxiety, stress, alertness, cognition
- Promote emotional insight and mood balancing
- Enhance sleep quality and relaxation response
- Reduce agitation, anger, fatigue, brain fog

Olfactory Effects

Aromas of essential oils stimulate the limbic region and olfactory nerves, eliciting reflex responses:

- Trigger neurotransmitters like serotonin that mediate mood and stress
- Influence the hormonal system responsible for cortisol, melatonin, and more
- Increase immune defense production of disease-fighting compounds
- Modulate the autonomic system to reduce fight-or-flight response

Energetic Effects

Essential oils' life force and plant consciousness resonate at higher vibrational levels that can directly rebalance human subtle energetic fields through:

- Chakra balancing to energize spiritual connection points
- Meridian stimulation to unblock chi flow for vitality
- Aura cleansing to dispel negativity and nurture inner light
- Meditative centering and mindfulness to cultivate inner peace

These multifaceted actions make aromatherapy a truly holistic and comprehensive natural healing system.

Origins of Aromatherapy in Ancient Civilizations

The origins of aromatherapy stretch back over 6,000 years, with extensive use of aromatic plant oils documented in ancient Egypt, China, India, Greece and Rome. Essential oils served therapeutic, spiritual and ceremonial purposes in early societies across the world:

Ancient Egypt

- The earliest evidence of distillation used oils in medicine, mummification,

Ancient India

- Ayurveda elaborately prescribed aromatherapy massage and oils for health

Ancient China

- Traditional Chinese medicine utilized aromatherapy oils like camphor, sandalwood,

Ancient Greece & Rome

- Greeks learned distillation techniques from Egypt, and Romans adopted practices.
- Medical texts documented distillation methods and health uses of oils

Indigenous cultures also used aromatic barks, resins and flowers ceremonially. Across early civilizations, essential oils were prized for wellness and ritual.

Aromatherapy Evolution from Ancient Times to Modern Era

The history of aromatherapy has evolved over thousands of years since ancient times, with a growing understanding of distillation, therapeutic properties and clinical applications:

Middle Ages

Distillation techniques appeared in alchemy and folk medicine texts but were often kept secret.

Early 20th Century

French chemist Rene-Maurice Gattefosse coined the term "aromatherapie" after using lavender oil to heal a burn.

1920s-40s

Gattefosse published seminal research on essential oils; Valnet used oils for injured soldiers in WWII.

1950s–1970s

Scientific studies expanded. Marguerite Maury opened the first aromatherapy clinic in London in 1964.

1980s-90s

Popularity surged as aromatherapy was embraced as a holistic healing technique.

Today

Aromatherapy continues to grow as a gentle, effective form of integrative medicine, drawing upon ancient plant wisdom.

CHAPTER 3

METHODS OF EXTRACTION

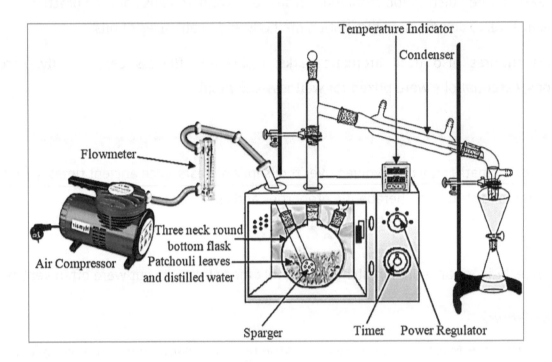

Essential oils are highly concentrated plant extracts that capture the aroma, flavor and therapeutic properties of their botanical sources. Producing these aromatic plant oils requires specialized extraction methods that carefully separate the volatile plant compounds from other elements of the plant material. This chapter provides an in-depth look at the various extraction processes used to obtain essential oils, including steam distillation, solvent extraction, cold pressing, supercritical CO2 extraction, and more. We will explore the procedures, equipment, advantages and disadvantages of each method.

Steam Distillation

The most common method for essential oil extraction is steam distillation. This involves using steam to carry volatile plant compounds like terpenes and phenylpropanoids away from plant material to condense the aromatic phytochemicals into an essential oil.

Steam distillation equipment consists of stainless steel still with a heat source, essential oil separator, condenser and collection vessel. Plant material is placed in the still, and the still is sealed and filled with steam. As the internal environment heats up, pockets of essential oils stored within the plant are freed and evaporate.

The steam and freed essential oil compounds travel up a distillation tube and reach a condenser, where the steam liquefies. This mixes the water and essential oils, but the oils, being hydrophobic, rise up through a separator into a collection vessel where the pure essential oil accumulates.

Water distillates containing trace amounts of essential oils are drawn off separately and may be cohobated or redistilled to recapture any remaining essential oils. What remains in the still after distillation is the aqueous plant hydrolate or hydrosol that contains plant acids, phytochemicals and water-soluble fractions.

The extraction time and temperature must be optimized for each plant species to maximize essential oil yields and preserve delicate aromatic compounds. Common oils extracted via steam distillation include lavender, peppermint, eucalyptus, tea tree, rosemary, lemon and frankincense.

Advantages of steam distillation include efficient extraction of leafy or woody plant materials at a relatively low cost. However, the high heat can damage heat-sensitive constituents in some plants. Steam distillation is less successful for plants containing high amounts of waxes, resins or bulky molecules.

Solvent Extraction

Solvent extraction employs organic solvents such as petroleum ether, methane, ethanol or hexane to extract essential oils from plant materials. During this process, plant material soaks in the organic solvent, enabling the solvent to dissolve and accumulate the plant's fixed oils along with the essential oil fragrance and therapeutic compounds.

The plant material is then filtered out, leaving a solution of the solvent mixed with the plant oils. The essential oils are separated from the fixed vegetable oils through evaporation of the solvent via vacuum or distillation techniques. The solvent can then be recovered and reused, though trace amounts usually remain in the oils. These solvent residues make the safety and purity of solvent-extracted oils questionable.

Solvent extraction is used to produce floral absolutes for perfumes but is problematic for therapeutic essential oils. While it does yield a wide range of plant compounds with high aromatic quality, traces of neurotoxic solvents like hexane can remain in absolutes. Harsher solvents like benzene can also be used. For these reasons, as well as high costs, solvent extraction is decreasing as safer and more efficient methods become popular.

Cold Pressing

Cold pressing is commonly used to extract citrus essential oils like lemon, sweet orange, bergamot, mandarin, grapefruit and lime. No heat is applied during this method. Instead, citrus rinds or peels are mechanically pressed to rupture the essential oil sacs and squeeze out the oils.

There are two techniques used for cold pressing. The Ecuelle à Piquer process involves pressing whole trimmed fruit between concave metal cups with sharp protruding spikes that pierce the peel, releasing essential oils. The more modern centrifugal pressing technique spins whole fruit or peels against paddles inside a centrifugal machine to rupture the oil glands. The expelled citrus oils, juices and other liquids are centrifugally separated, with the water-immiscible essential oil layer pooled off for collection.

Cold pressing is a straightforward, solvent-free process that preserves many fragile aroma compounds. It yields relatively low amounts of essential oil. The fresh, luminous citrus oils produced are widely used in aromatherapy, perfumery and cleaning formulas. No redistillation or solvents are involved, maximizing the retention of delicate aromatic compounds. The limitation is that it only applies to oils from the thick rinds of citrus fruits.

Supercritical Carbon Dioxide Extraction

Supercritical carbon dioxide (CO2) extraction is a modern method gaining popularity for selectively extracting aromatic plant compounds to produce very high-quality essential oils. It uses carbon dioxide liquified under pressure, which acquires enhanced solvent properties.

Plant material is placed into a chamber, and pressurized CO2 is pumped in as a solvent. The pressure and temperature are carefully manipulated, taking the CO2 into its "supercritical" state. This gives it excellent solvent power to dissolve and extract the delicate aromatic essential oil compounds.

Once extraction completes, the pressure is reduced, and CO2 evaporates, leaving behind the extracted material with no residual solvents. The CO2 can then be recaptured and reused. CO2 extraction is performed with expensive equipment and specialist oversight. It has versatile selectivity and protects vulnerable compounds. Oils like rose, jasmine, vanilla, hops and ginseng are effectively extracted using this method. No heat or solvents risk damaging the precious ingredients.

Expression

Expression is a simple approach used almost exclusively for citrus oils. The outermost peel of citrus fruits contains specialized glandular oil sacs holding the aromatic essential oils. By mechanically pressing the rind, these sacs rupture and release the essential oil.

Hand expression involves manually pressing the citrus peels and blotting the tiny droplets of expelled oils. Small-scale artisans may use this technique. More often, motorized citrus presses are employed. They mechanically squeeze and grind the peels while spraying water to collect the released essential oils.

However, expression yields low amounts of essential oil with less complete extraction than cold pressing methods. Hand expression also risks discouragement when little oil materializes after much effort. So, expression is limited to small artisanal producers or used as a precursor to cold pressing.

Enfleurage

Enfleurage is a labor-intensive method used to extract essential oils from delicate flower petals like jasmine, tuberose and rose. These flowers yield trace amounts of essential oil through distillation. Enfleurage maximizes the aromatic compounds extracted by using fats as fixatives.

Glass plates are coated evenly with highly refined, odorless vegetable fats or oils, like grapeseed or jojoba. Fresh blossoms are laid atop the fat, and the glass plates are stacked tightly. Every 12-24 hours, the faded blossoms are replaced with a new layer of fresh petals.

After several weeks or months of replacing flowers, the fats are completely saturated with the flower essences. Alcohol is then used to dissolve the fragrant fatty oils. The alcohol evaporates away via distillation, leaving behind a wax-like mass called concrete. Further processing with alcohol yields the final floral "absolute."

Enfleurage is still used in fine perfume production but rarely for aromatherapy oils. It yields very small quantities – thousands of flower petals produce just a few milliliters of essential oil. The prohibitive costs and labor make enfleurage extremely limited. But it does create concentrated extracts with unparalleled aromatic quality.

Fermentation

Certain plant materials can undergo fermentation to separate aromatic compounds into an essential oil. Fermentation involves microbial activity that metabolizes and transforms organic substances into alcohols, organic acids, gases and other products.

Plant materials are washed, chopped and soaked in water to form a mash. Yeast, bacteria, enzymes or fungal cultures are introduced, and the fermentation process begins. As fermentation progresses, heat and enzymes break down plant cells, releasing volatiles. Active fermenting takes place for anywhere from a few days to over a month.

Once complete, the fermented mash is steam-distilled to vaporize and collect the aromatic essential oils. Oils extracted via fermentation include jasmine, vetiver, patchouli, spices like black pepper, and birch. The resulting oils have distinct terroir from microbial metabolites influencing aroma profiles. However, consistency and quality control are challenges.

Resin Tapping

Certain plants naturally excrete aromatic resins or oleoresins from wounds in their bark. Collecting these resins can provide essential oils called oleogums with intense fragrances. Birch trees, pine trees, styrax and members of the Boswellia and Bursera genera produce valuable medicinal resins.

In resin tapping, cuts are made into the bark to initiate resin production, directing the flow into collection vessels. Holes may be drilled into the trunks or slashes made into the bark. Cuts are not too deep to maintain tree health. The resin can be tapped multiple times as it regenerates.

Hand tapping is slow and laborious. More efficient techniques, like using vacuum pumps to suck out oleoresin without large gashes, are often employed for sustainable harvesting. Once collected, the resins first need solvent extraction to remove rubber, foliage and impurities. The resins then undergo steam distillation to isolate the essential oils.

Key oleogum oils produced through resin tapping include frankincense, myrrh, pine, styrax and copaiba balsam. This method provides Middle Eastern and African oils that have been prized since antiquity for spiritual and therapeutic uses.

Other Methods

Some less common extraction methods also exist. Maceration involves soaking plant material in warm oil to leach out aromatic compounds. Pomade production uses animal fat soaked with fragrant herbs or flowers as a perfume fixative. Organic vegetable oil infused with lemon or orange peels makes a cold-pressed peel oil.

While simple and natural, these techniques yield oils with lower levels of desired volatile aromatics. So essential oils are often subsequently solvent extracted or distilled from the fats, plant oils or pomades via a co-distillation process. This allows capturing higher amounts of active essential oil constituents compared with just relying on maceration or enfleurage alone.

No single extraction method is ideal or applicable to all plants. The production process varies depending on the plant source and desired essential oil. Mastering multiple techniques allows professional aromatherapists to work with a diverse palette of custom-crafted essential oils.

Steam Distillation Procedure

Steam distillation is the most common method for essential oil extraction, used with leafy and woody plants like lavender, eucalyptus, rosemary and tea trees. Here is an overview of the steam distillation process:

- Chopped plant material is placed into a still along with water
- Still is sealed and heated, often via an external steam jacket or internal coils
- Steam carries volatile compounds through a distillation tube upward
- The tube leads to the condenser, where steam liquefies, releasing aromatics
- Mixed water and essential oils flow into the separation vessel
- Oils float to the top due to their hydrophobic nature and are siphoned off
- The remaining water distillate contains trace oils (hydrosols)
- Plant material left in still is spent botanical residue (pomace)
- Distillation time/temperature optimized for each plant species
- Yield maximized while preserving delicate aromatic compounds

Properly done, steam distillation efficiently extracts essential oils with pressure, temperature and duration tailored to the plant source. It optimally balances yield, completeness and preservation of fragile constituents.

Solvent Extraction Methods and Concerns

Solvent extraction employs organic solvents to dissolve and extract essential oils and aromatic compounds from plants. Common techniques include:

- Maceration - Plant soaks in hot solvent, filtered out
- Percolation - Solvent drips through packed plant material
- Distillation - Plant soaked in solvent, then distilled off
- Enfleurage - Plant matter infuses odorless fats and alcohol used to extract

Popular solvents include hexane, methanol, ethanol, benzene and petroleum ether due to efficacy and low costs. However, toxicity concerns arise with traces of neurotoxic hexane, carcinogenic benzene and other harsh solvents potentially remaining in finished oils intended for aromatherapy use. Even "food-grade" hexane can contain up to 1% benzene. Solvent extraction is decreasing in popularity due to safety issues. Safer approaches like supercritical CO2 extraction are becoming preferable when higher costs allow.

CHAPTER 4
SAFETY GUIDELINES AND PRECAUTIONS

Essential oils are highly concentrated, biologically active plant extracts that must be used with care and caution. Following proper safety guidelines is critical when working with these powerful botanical compounds. Certain oils require particular precautions regarding dosage, dilution, contraindications, sensitization risks, phototoxic potential and more. This chapter will provide a comprehensive overview of essential oil safety considerations, including appropriate usage, storage, toxicity data, contraindications, drug interactions, and safe handling procedures. We will also explore safety guidelines for special populations like children, seniors and pregnant women.

General Safety Guidelines

When used correctly, essential oils can be incorporated into daily life safely. However, as concentrated plant extracts, oils can cause adverse reactions if misused. Here are some key safety guidelines:

- Educate yourself thoroughly on safety procedures for each oil
- Research contraindications for the health conditions you have
- Perform a skin patch test to check for allergic reactions before regular use
- Always dilute essential oils prior to topical use with a suitable carrier oil
- Use lower dilutions on children; 1% or less is recommended
- Avoid certain oils during pregnancy, especially in 1st trimester
- Check for drug interactions before combining oils with medications
- Keep bottles tightly closed and away from children's reach
- Never ingest oils unless under the guidance of an aromatherapy professional

Following these common-sense precautions and the specific safety data for each essential oil will help prevent adverse reactions. Consult a certified aromatherapist or healthcare provider for personalized safety guidance.

Dosage and Dilution Guidelines

Essential oils are highly concentrated plant extracts and must be diluted before use in most cases.

Typical dilution guidelines:

Topical - For adults, 2-5% is standard (2-5 drops per teaspoon of carrier), up to 10% for acute issues. 1% or less for children.

Baths - Generally, 3-7 drops per adult bath, 10 drops max. 1 drop max per bath for children.

Room diffusers - Follow manufacturer maximum, usually around 20 drops per 200ml water capacity.

Inhalation - 2-4 drops in an inhaler or diffuser, less for children. Avoid direct inhalation.

Internal use - ONLY under the strict guidance of a professional aromatherapist or doctor.

Photosensitizing Oils

Some essential oils contain furocoumarins and other phototoxic compounds that can cause severe burns, blisters or pigmentation issues when exposed to UV light. They include:

- Citrus oils: bergamot, lemon, lime, grapefruit, bitter orange
- Angelica root, rue, cumin, verbena, ginger, dill

Photosensitizing oils should be avoided or minimized, never used at over 2% dilution, and completely avoided for sun exposure. They can still be suitable for diffused or topical use at proper dilutions if not exposed to direct sunlight.

Contraindications and Special Populations

Those who are pregnant, nursing, elderly, have chronic illnesses or are taking prescription medicines should take extra care with essential oil use due to increased sensitization risks. It's best to first consult an aromatherapist or doctor knowledgeable in essential oils for guidance on contraindicated oils and safety precautions. General considerations include:

Pregnancy

Many oils should be avoided in 1st trimester when organogenesis occurs, and absorption risks exist. Use the lowest possible dilutions.

Infants & Young Children

Extremely low dilutions were used, 0.5-1% or less. Many oils are contraindicated until age 3.

Elderly

Dilutions on the lower side due to increased skin sensitivity and medication use. Lighter, uplifting scents are often preferred.

Chronic Illnesses

Oils that reduce blood clotting, lower blood sugar/pressure, worsen hormone-sensitive cancers or cause neurological reactions require caution.

Drug Interactions

Oils may increase absorption or change the metabolism of prescription medications, increasing the risk of side effects.

Essential Oil Allergies and Sensitivities

Always do a skin patch test before regular use of any essential oil. Allergic reactions and acquired sensitization can develop over time with repeated exposure. Discontinue use immediately if any irritation develops. Lavender, ylang-ylang, lemongrass, tea tree and citrus oils most often cause sensitization. Those with allergies or skin conditions are at greater risk. Sensitization is unpredictable but reversible if the offending oil is avoided.

Adulterated or Synthetic Oils

Using pure, authentic, unadulterated essential oils is vital for safety. Synthetic nature-identical oils, extended oils diluted with solvents and oils adulterated with synthetic chemicals can cause allergic reactions and toxicity. Source from reputable suppliers who provide GC/MS spec reports. If an oil seems irritating or does not smell true, it may contain synthetics or adulterants.

Internal Use Precautions

Ingesting essential oils carries more risks than topical applications and is not recommended for home use without professional supervision. Potential dangers include mucous membrane irritation, toxicity to the liver and kidneys from metabolizing oil compounds, seizures, breathing issues, slowed heart rate and internal bleeding if oils that prolong clotting time are ingested. Never ingest any oil not approved for food grade. Work with an aromatherapist trained in internal protocols to minimize risks.

Essential Oil Safety Data

Specific essential oils have unique safety considerations and potential side effects. Reviewing detailed safety data for each oil helps identify proper usage and contraindications. Key safety information to look for includes:

- Botanical species, any adulteration risks
- Route of administration guidelines
- Maximum dermal use level, any photosensitivity
- Potential skin, mucous membrane or respiratory irritancy
- Children and elderly usage cautions
- Drug interactions, medical cautions
- Toxicology data like LD50, dermal toxicity, chronic exposure effects
- Contraindications for conditions like pregnancy, cancer, liver/kidney disease

These parameters provide critical usage guidance. Safety can be enhanced by selecting oils from reputable suppliers who disclose such data.

Essential Oil Storage to Maintain Safety

Properly storing essential oils maximizes their safety and shelf life:

- Keep bottles tightly sealed to limit oxidation and evaporation
- Store in stable, moderate temperature conditions; avoid heat/light exposure

- Do not refrigerate oils, which can promote condensation issues
- Use oils within shelf life period; citrus and pine oils have shorter lifespan
- Transfer a small portion for active use, and keep the bulk oil supply sealed
- Avoid cross-contamination by never sharing droppers between bottles

Proper storage limits damage or degradation over time to help oils retain therapeutic potency and safe chemistry.

Safe Handling of Essential Oils

Essential oils can irritate the skin and eyes. Take care when handling undiluted oils:

- Wash hands after handling essential oils
- Work in well-ventilated space; do not breathe oils directly
- Wear nitrile gloves if you have sensitive skin
- Never apply undiluted oils directly on the skin; dilute first
- Avoid contact with eyes, mucous membranes
- Do not ingest oils unless under professional guidance
- Keep bottles tightly capped when not in use
- Store out of reach of children and pets

With common-sense handling, essential oil use can be enjoyable and safe.

Essential Oil Toxicity and Side Effects

Essential oils contain hundreds of bioactive compounds that can cause side effects in some individuals, especially at improper doses. Potential side effects include:

- Skin irritation, allergic reactions, sensitization - Often due to oxidation or adulteration
- Phototoxic reactions - From furocoumarins reacting to sunlight
- Respiratory irritation - Pepper-like sting if inhaled directly due to phenols
- Mucous membrane irritation - Pain sores from contact with undiluted oils
- Cardiac effects - Change in heart rate and blood pressure from certain oils
- Neurotoxicity - Dizziness, seizures, coma from an overdose of oils like camphor, eucalyptus, sage
- Liver and kidney toxicity - Damage from ingesting/metabolizing some oil compounds
- Medication interactions - Altering absorption, metabolism, and effects of prescription drugs

Safety becomes a greater concern for at-risk groups like children, the elderly and pregnant women, as well as those with chronic illnesses. Proper usage guidelines, dosing and contraindication avoidance minimize the risks of serious side effects.

Essential Oil First Aid

Accidental exposure to undiluted essential oils may require a first aid response:

- If spilled on the skin - Wash the area with soap and water. Avoid spreading oil further.
- Suppose splashed in eyes - Flush eyes with cool water for 15 minutes. Seek medical care if irritation persists. Do not rub your eyes.
- Suppose ingested - Drink milk or water to dilute. Do NOT induce vomiting. Call Poison Control if ingested.
- If inhaled - Move to fresh air. Apply Vicks VapoRub under the nose to help stop inhalation.
- For severe reactions like seizures, irregular heartbeat or breathing issues, seek immediate medical help. Prompt first aid can lessen adverse reactions until proper medical treatment is received.

BOOK 2

ESSENTIAL OILS FOR PHYSICAL HEALTH AND WELLNESS

BOOSTING IMMUNITY

(IMMUNE-BOOSTING OILS, INHALATION TECHNIQUES)

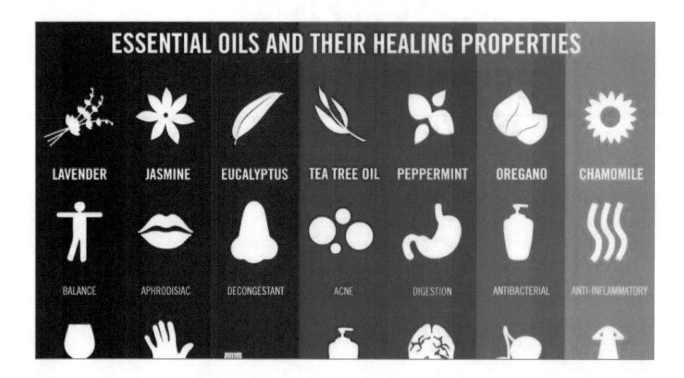

Essential oils provide a holistic way to support immune function and help defend against pathogens. Certain oils contain compounds shown to stimulate white blood cell production, battle viruses and bacteria, reduce inflammation, fight fungal overgrowth, and enhance specific and non-specific immunity. This chapter will explore the top immune-boosting essential oils, their mechanisms of action, and effective techniques for using aromatherapy to optimize immune response.

How Essential Oils Support Immunity

Essential oils uplift immunity through several mechanisms:

Antimicrobial Effects

Many essential oils exhibit direct antimicrobial actions against viruses, bacteria, fungi and parasites. Oils contain terpenes, phenols, aldehydes and esters that can rupture microbial cell walls and disrupt reproductive cycles and other cellular functions. Popular antimicrobial oils include oregano, thyme, lemon, tea tree, eucalyptus, clove and cinnamon. Diffusing these oils can cleanse ambient air of potentially harmful microbes.

Anti-Inflammatory Actions

Compounds in oils like chamomile, lavender, frankincense and clary sage help regulate inflammatory pathways on a cellular level. They balance pro- and anti-inflammatory prostaglandins and cytokines to reduce excessive inflammation while still allowing a normal immune response. This modulation prevents a dangerous cytokine storm yet still supports microbial clearance.

Immune Cell Stimulation

Essential oils spur the activity of immune system cells like lymphocytes, phagocytes, and natural killer cells, which target pathogens. Oils that boost lymphocyte production include sandalwood, frankincense, Ravensara, lemon, oregano and mountain savory. This arms the immune system for heightened microbial threats.

Lymphatic Drainage Support

The lymphatic system filters toxins, waste and pathogens from tissues. Drainage slows during illness. Essential oils help stimulate lymphatic circulation when used in lymphatic massage techniques. This improves immune cell trafficking, waste removal, and fluid balance.

Antioxidant Effects

The free radical scavenging activity of oils helps protect cells from oxidative damage caused by microbial toxins and inflammatory immune chemicals. This preserves their function in defending the body against pathogens. Bergamot, clove, thyme, oregano and cinnamon oils have potent antioxidant capacity.

Top Immune-Boosting Oils and Recipes

Many essential oils help strengthen immunity. The following stand out for their broad actions supporting immune health:

Oregano

Powerfully antimicrobial, antiviral and antibacterial due to thymol and carvacrol content. It is also anti-inflammatory and antioxidant. Add several drops to a bath or diffuse.

Thyme

Stimulates white blood cell production while battling microbes. Use in mouthwashes and steam inhalation.

Eucalyptus

Decongestant, antiviral, antimicrobial. Opens airways and clears mucus during respiratory infections. Diffuse or inhale via steam tent.

Cinnamon Bark

Strong antifungal, antibacterial, and antiviral oil, especially against antibiotic-resistant strains. Use topically or gargle diluted oil.

Lemon

Stimulates lymph drainage and white blood cell production. Add lemon oil to tea daily as an immune tonic.

Frankincense

Boosts lymphocyte production and combats inflammation. Add to a diffuser for long-term immune support.

Tea Tree Oil

Broad-spectrum antimicrobial properties battle viral, bacterial and fungal infections topically and via inhalation.

Clove Bud

It is one of the strongest antiviral and antimicrobial oils due to its eugenol content. Use for acute infections.

Rosemary

Anti-inflammatory, antioxidant, and antimicrobial actions support healthy immune responses. Diffuse with orange to lift the mood.

Bergamot

Contains anti-inflammatory flavonoids that also increase leukocyte migration. Uplifting scent promotes relaxation.

Essential Oil Application Methods for Immune Support

There are several techniques for effectively using essential oils to boost immunity:

Diffusion Volatile oils dispersed into the air are inhaled and absorbed into the lungs and bloodstream, where they exert antiviral, antibacterial and immune-stimulating effects systemically. Oils can also sanitize ambient air of airborne pathogens when diffused. Diffuse continuously during seasonal health threats or for several hours daily to maintain immune support.

Steam Inhalation

Inhaling moist air infused with essential oils brings antimicrobial, expectorant and decongestant vapors directly to the lungs, sinuses and respiratory tract. Add oils like eucalyptus, peppermint, pine, melaleuca or thyme to a bowl of hot water. Place a towel over your head and carefully breathe the vapors for 5-10 minutes as tolerated.

Topical Application

Essential oils penetrate the skin and underlying mucosa rapidly. Applying immune-boosting oils diluted in carrier oil helps activate circulation and immune defenses in the area while absorbing into the bloodstream for wider effects. Rub oil blends on lymph nodes, chest, sinuses or reflexology immune system points.

Lymphatic Massage

Lymphatic massage with essential oils stimulates cleansing lymph flow throughout the body. Use light strokes towards the heart along lymph pathways. Add oils like grapefruit, lemon and cypress to massage oil. Perform daily when fighting infection.

Baths

Adding immune-boosting oils to a warm bath allows respiratory and skin absorption as well as relaxation benefits. The heat further decongests bronchial and sinus passages. Recommended oils are eucalyptus, pine, melaleuca, lavender and marjoram.

Oral Use

While ingestion is not generally recommended, some gentle immune oils may be taken internally under the guidance of an aromatherapist. Oils taken in capsules or drops can provide direct antimicrobial action and immune stimulation systemically. Only use very mild oils like lemon, oregano, and frankincense short term.

Pairing essential oil techniques with adequate sleep, hydration and nutrition further optimizes immune response. Consistency is key for lasting immune support.

Boosting Immunity in Children and Elderly

Boosting immunity becomes even more important in vulnerable populations like the very young and elderly. Children and seniors are at increased risk of severe infection due to developing or weakened immune systems. However, care must be taken with potency and safety precautions in these groups. Here are tips for using essential oils to safely improve immunity for children and the elderly:

Children

- Use gentle oils like lavender, frankincense, lemon, tea tree
- Extremely low dilutions used – 0.25% to 1%
- Avoid potentially toxic oils like pine, cinnamon, clove,
- Minimize skin applications, focus more on diffusion
- Monitor closely for any reactions or sensitization

Elderly

- Avoid immune-suppressing oils like clary sage, chamomile,
- Use mild oils that stimulate immunity like lemon, orange, frankincense
- Apply topically to reflex points and lymph nodes to activate circulation
- Diffuse antiviral oils during infectious disease outbreaks
- Support with hydration, nutrition and sleep

The fragrant, uplifting aromas of immune-supporting oils help create a positive atmosphere of healing, comfort and strength. Essential oils give caregivers a practical way to enhance immune response and resilience in those most vulnerable.

Essential Oil Inhalation for Immunity

Inhaling diffused essential oils allows direct respiratory absorption and widespread delivery throughout the body. Babies, children, adults and the elderly can benefit without the risks of applying oils topically.

Direct inhalation also allows antimicrobial oils to protect against airborne viruses and germs. Here are tips for boosting immunity through inhalation:

Diffuser Use

- Add immune oils like eucalyptus, tea tree, thyme, oregano, frankincense
- Run diffuser continuously in high-traffic public areas during health threats
- Use ultrasonic cool mist diffusers for the longest aromatic diffusion
- Follow manufacturer guidelines and essential oil safety precautions

Steam Inhalation

- Create a steam tent by leaning over a bowl of hot water with a towel draped overhead.
- Carefully add oils like eucalyptus, pine, peppermint, melaleuca
- Inhale vapors for 5-10 minutes as tolerated to thin mucus, fight infection
- Keep eyes closed to prevent irritation

Direct Inhalation

- Apply 2-3 drops of gentle oil like lavender or tea tree to a cotton ball
- Inhale lightly from a cotton ball, keeping ~6 inches away from the nose
- Use less oil for children and avoid direct inhalation

For acute respiratory infections, inhale antiviral oils multiple times per day. For prevention, more occasional inhalation supports immune health without sensitizing airways. Inhalation allows versatile, convenient immune support for all ages.

CHAPTER 2

RESPIRATORY HEALTH
(CONGESTION RELIEF, SINUS SUPPORT)

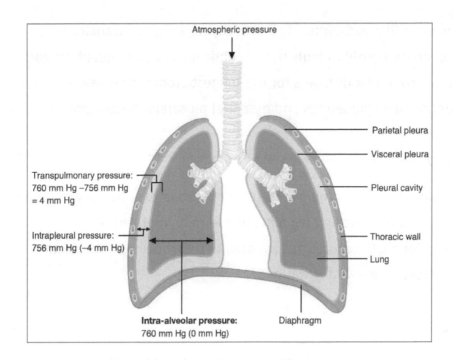

Essential oils provide natural relief for many respiratory complaints, including coughs, colds, congestion, sore throat, bronchitis, sinus issues, and respiratory infections. Oils contain volatile compounds that are readily inhaled into the lungs, bronchioles, sinuses and throat, where they exert antimicrobial, expectorant, anti-inflammatory, bronchodilatory, mucolytic and soothing effects. This chapter explores the most beneficial respiratory oils, along with recipes and techniques for using aromatherapy to optimize respiratory health and provide congestion relief.

Essential Oil Benefits for Respiratory Health

Here are some of the evidence-based benefits that essential oils offer for respiratory complaints:

Congestion Relief Mentholated oils like eucalyptus, peppermint and camphor open constricted airways and thin mucus secretions and stimulate coughing out of congestion when inhaled or diffused.

Sore Throat Soothing Analgesic and anesthetizing oils like clove, myrrh, oregano and thyme numb throat pain, reduce inflammation and fight viral causes of pharyngitis when used topically or gargled.

Cough Suppression Sedating, throat-coating oils like marjoram, spike lavender, helichrysum and frankincense help suppress dry, unproductive coughs. Expectorant oils like pine, cypress and benzoin reduce wet coughs.

Anti-Inflammatory Effects Lavender, German chamomile, helichrysum and other anti-inflammatory oils help curb excessive sinus inflammation, bronchial swelling and respiratory irritation.

Antimicrobial Properties Oils like oregano, melaleuca, lemon eucalyptus and cinnamon exhibit direct antiviral, antibacterial and antifungal effects against respiratory pathogens.

Respiratory Tract Cleansing Mucolytic oils like pine, eucalyptus, thyme and hyssop thin mucus secretions while soothing oils like marjoram reduce muscular spasms for easier expectoration.

Bronchodilation Eucalyptus oils relax the bronchial smooth muscle to open airways and increase air flow. Peppermint likewise cools and dilates passages.

With widespread use for coughs, colds, flu and congestion, aromatic plant oils offer safe, multidimensional respiratory relief without drowsiness, side effects or overuse concerns of OTC medications.

Best Essential Oils for Respiratory Support

Many essential oils benefit respiratory health. The following stand out as the most versatile for various respiratory complaints:

Eucalyptus

Potent decongestant, antiviral and expectorant. Opens airways, thins mucus and relieves coughs, colds and congestion.

Peppermint

Menthol cools and dilates airways and clears congestion. Alleviates sinus pressure, coughs, and sore throat. Invigorating.

Thyme

Powerful antibacterial and antiviral. Disinfects lungs and stops infection spread. Reduces coughs, bronchitis, and chest congestion.

Oregano

Strong antiviral and antibacterial actions fight respiratory infections. Useful for sore throats, coughs, sinusitis, and bronchitis.

Lemon

Aids respiratory tract cleansing and supports immune response against pathogens. Add to water, tea or diffuse.

Tea Tree

Broad-spectrum antimicrobial properties fight viral, bacterial and fungal lung infections. Reduces asthma triggers.

Pine

The balsamic aroma helps expel mucus secretions. Antiviral and decongestant for coughs, colds, and flu.

Marjoram

Soothes sore throat and suppresses coughs. Relieves chest tightness and respiratory muscle spasms.

Frankincense

Anti-inflammatory, immunostimulant and lung tonic. Clears lungs while reducing asthma attacks and allergies.

Cypress

Astringent and decongestant properties benefit chronic coughs, bronchitis, and whooping cough in dilution.

Using the right oils for each respiratory complaint through diffused inhalation or topical methods provides effective, natural congestion relief and respiratory support.

Application Methods for Respiratory Relief

Essential oils can be applied in various ways to achieve respiratory benefits:

Steam Inhalation

Inhaling moist vapors directly brings oils' aromatic compounds into the sinuses, bronchial passages, lungs and throat for localized effects. Add oils to hot water and breathe deeply under a towel tent.

Diffusers

Oils like eucalyptus and tea trees dispersed in room air provide constant decongestant, antimicrobial protection. Cool mist diffusers avoid heat degradation of constituents.

Chest Rubs

Rubbing congestion-busting oil blends diluted in a carrier oil directly on the chest, neck and throat allows absorption while inhaling vapors up close.

Gargles and Sore Throat Sprays

Gargling with oils like oregano, clove, thyme and lemon reduces throat inflammation, pain and infection while their volatiles are released into the throat and nasal passages.

Humidifiers and Vaporizers

Adding oils to humidifier water allows heat and moisture to vaporize oils. The warm steam tent effect irrigates sinus passages and lungs with aromatic compounds.

Nasal/Sinus Inhalation

Inhaling oil vapors directly into the nasal cavities or sinuses allows concentrated benefits. Care must be taken to avoid irritating delicate tissues.

Baths

Dispersing oils into hot bath water provides full-body absorption and inhalation effects. Asthmatics should be used cautiously as heat can trigger airflow limitation in some.

Topical Chest Application

Applying diluted oils like eucalyptus, rosemary and frankincense over lung reflex points on the chest and back allows absorption while inhaling close vapors.

Oral Administration

Taking extremely dilute oils like lemon internally provides direct respiratory tissue anti-inflammatory and antimicrobial effects. Requires professional guidance.

Air Purification

Cold air diffusers with oils like lemon, pine and tea tree filter and sanitize room air of microbes and allergens.

Using the right method for each condition allows for maximizing relief. Inhalation methods provide the fastest aromatherapeutic benefits.

Essential Oil Steam Inhalation

Steam inhalation brings the direct respiratory benefits of essential oils into warm, moist air that effectively transfers the volatile compounds into nasal passages, throat, sinuses and lungs. To perform steam inhalation:

- Fill a large bowl with freshly boiled water, remove from heat
- Drape a towel over the head to form a tent trapping the steam
- Carefully add 3-7 drops of essential oil like eucalyptus or mint
- Keep eyes closed and breathe deeply for 5-10 minutes
- Can repeat 2-3 times daily as needed for congestion

Tips:

- Adjust the oil amount based on aroma strength
- Those with asthma or lung disease should be cautious with steam
- Keep eyes closed and discontinue if irritation develops
- Use 100% natural, therapeutic-grade essential oils
- Clean oils may be reused for up to a week if stored properly

The warm moisture softens mucus secretions while the aromatic compounds penetrate and open airways. Oils like peppermint, pine, thyme and oregano provide added antiviral and antibacterial protection. Use steam inhalation at first signs of respiratory infection or congestion for rapid relief.

Essential Oils for Coughs and Sore Throats

Coughs represent the body's protective reflex to clear irritants or secretions from the respiratory tract. Sore throats signal infection or inflammation. Essential oils alleviate both:

For dry coughs, use oils that suppress the coughing reflex:

- Marjoram, helichrysum, spike lavender

For wet, productive coughs, use expectorant oils:

- Pine, eucalyptus, cypress

For sore throats, use analgesic and anesthetizing oils:

- Lavender, tea tree, thyme, lemon, clove

Throat spray recipes:

- Add 1 drop of clove, thyme, and oregano essential oils to a 2 oz spray bottle filled with water
- Shake before use. Spray 2-4 times onto the back of the throat as needed

Oral rinse/gargle recipe:

- Add 1 drop of lemon, lavender, melaleuca essential oils to 1 cup of warm water
- Gargle for 30 seconds as needed to reduce throat tickle, pain, and inflammation

Other tips:

- Take expectorant oils internally only under professional guidance
- Diffuse cough-suppressing oils at night to allow rest
- Inhale cough-reducing oils before cough-provoking triggers

Rather than suppressing coughs, essential oils treat the root causes – like infection, irritation and excess mucus. A combination approach brings multidimensional relief safely and effectively.

Congestion Relief for Sinusitis

Sinusitis causes uncomfortable congestion, facial pressure, headache and postnasal drip due to inflamed sinuses. Inhaling the following essential oils helps provide relief:

Eucalyptus oil

Potent decongestant, anti-inflammatory, and antimicrobial effects. Opens passages.

Peppermint oil

Cools inflamed tissues and clears blockages with menthol content.

Oregano oil

Strong anti-infective properties fight bacterial causes of sinus infections.

Frankincense oil

Anti-inflammatory boswellic acids reduce sinus swelling and irritation.

Tea tree oil

Broad spectrum antimicrobial actions battle sinus infection.

Lavender oil

Soothes sinus pain and headaches associated with sinusitis.

Diffuse oils to inhale vapors. Steam inhalation also brings concentrated vapor into the sinuses. Massage diluted oils over sinus points on the nose, cheeks and forehead. For acute sinus infection, utilize oregano or thyme internally only under guidance.

Respiratory Health for Babies and Children

Coughs, colds, allergies and chest congestion frequently affect babies and children. Yet safety precautions must be taken when using essential oils on kids. Here are tips:

Age 0-2 years:

- No direct inhalation or topical use except under guidance
- Diffuse very gently in the bedroom away from the baby
- Oils like lavender, chamomile, frankincense

Age 2-6 years:

- Only gentle oil inhalation for short periods
- Topical use is still risky – only lightly diffuse
- Continue mild, soothing oils

Age 6-12 years:

- Begin diluted topical use on feet or chest
- Watch closely for skin reactions
- Low-concentration inhalation okay
- Use gentle oils like eucalyptus, tea tree, pine

Maximize diffused inhalation and minimize topical use. Use gentle oils at very low concentrations. Let kids self-limit exposure. Monitor closely and educate on proper usage to encourage mindful utilization.

Essential Oil Chest Rubs

Diluted essential oils applied to the chest provide respiratory relief through inhalation of vapors as well as absorption into underlying airways. To make a chest rub:

- Add 8-10 drops of essential oils per 1 ounce of carrier oil like coconut or jojoba oil
- Oils to use: eucalyptus, peppermint, pine, frankincense, thyme
- Rub a small amount gently onto the chest, neck and upper back
- Inhale vapors deeply
- Keep away from nostrils and eyes
- Store excess in an airtight container away from sunlight

The rub penetrates bronchial passages while vapors inhaled carry compounds deep into the lungs. This allows a direct route to clear congestion, fight infection, open airways, reduce inflammation and soothe tissues. An aromatic chest rub offers easy, rapid respiratory relief.

CHAPTER 3

NATURAL PAIN RELIEF

(ANTI-INFLAMMATORY OILS,
TOPICAL APPLICATIONS)

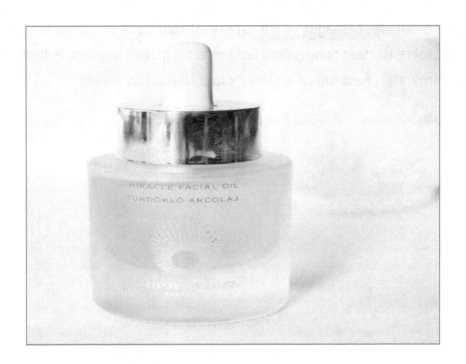

Essential oils provide a holistic alternative for relieving many types of pain, including muscle aches, headaches, joint pain, nerve pain, menstrual cramps, and post-operative pain. Anti-inflammatory, analgesic, antispasmodic and anesthetic compounds in the oils work through various mechanisms to safely reduce pain and inflammation when applied topically or inhaled. This chapter explores the most effective pain-relieving essential oils, along with recipes and techniques for natural, aromatherapeutic pain management.

Best Essential Oils for Pain Relief

Many essential oils have been studied for analgesic and anti-inflammatory effects. The most researched and versatile for pain relief include:

Lavender

Contains analgesics like linalool and linalyl acetate. Reduces muscle soreness, headache, joint and nerve pain.

Chamomile

Anti-inflammatory, anesthetic, muscle relaxant. Soothes headaches, muscle spasms, TMJ, and nerve pain.

Peppermint

Analgesic, cooling, anesthetic menthol relieves joint pain, headache, muscle aches, and neuralgia.

Wintergreen

Powerful analgesic similar to aspirin. Use for acute pain like headaches, arthritis, and tendinitis.

Rosemary

Analgesic, anti-inflammatory carnosol soothes muscle pain, sciatica, rheumatic pain, and headaches.

Eucalyptus

Stimulating, anti-inflammatory oil helps muscular aches, knee pain, arthritis, and neuropathy.

Helichrysum

Anti-inflammatory for nerve, muscle, rheumatic and migraine pain. Tissue regenerator.

Clary Sage

Antispasmodic relieves muscle cramps and spasms, menstrual pain, and stomach aches.

Frankincense

Potent anti-inflammatory, immunostimulant and analgesic for chronic pain and arthritis.

Marjoram

Analgesic, vasodilator, muscle relaxer used for headache, muscle spasms, cramps, TMJ.

Yarrow

Anti-inflammatory analgesic with natural pain-blocking chemicals used for wounds, arthritis, and tooth pain.

Essential Oil Recipes and Remedies for Pain

Essential oils can be used in various ways to achieve natural analgesia:

Headache Relief Rollerball Blend

- 10 drops peppermint essential oil
- 5 drops of lavender essential oil
- 2 drops of marjoram essential oil
- Fill a 10ml rollerball bottle with fractionated coconut oil
- Roll onto temples, forehead, neck and shoulders for headache pain

Muscle Relief Cream

- 2 drops rosemary, eucalyptus, wintergreen oils
- 1 tablespoon coconut oil
- Mix together and rub onto sore, stiff, spasming muscles

Arthritis and Joint Pain Oil

- 5 drops each wintergreen, peppermint, helichrysum, and frankincense oils
- 1 ounce carrier oil like jojoba or coconut
- Massage onto affected joints to reduce inflammation, swelling and stiffness

Nerve Pain Relief Compress

- Add 2 drops helichrysum and 5 drops chamomile oils to warm compress
- Apply to areas of nerve pain such as sciatica, neuropathy, shingles,

Menstrual Cramp Massage Oil

- 4 drops clary sage, lavender, and marjoram essential oils
- 1 tablespoon coconut carrier oil
- Gently massage over the lower abdomen and lower back

Post-Surgery Healing Spray

- 5 drops helichrysum, lavender, frankincense oils
- 1 ounce witch hazel hydrosol or distilled water
- Spray over incisions to promote healing and reduce pain

Diluted essential oils can be applied topically through massage, compresses, baths and therapeutic creams for effective, holistic pain relief. Certain gentle oils may also be taken internally under professional guidance for acute pain.

Essential Oil Massage for Pain

Massaging affected areas with diluted essential oils provides direct absorption of analgesic and anti-inflammatory compounds into muscles, joints and nerves while inhaling the aromatherapeutic vapors. Follow these steps:

1. Select appropriate essential oils for pain complaint
2. Dilute 4-8 drops of oils per ounce of carrier oil like coconut or jojoba
3. Apply a thin layer of the oil blend to the area of pain
4. Use light stroking motions, avoiding friction over inflamed regions
5. Focus on massaging tense, contracted muscles
6. Apply warm compresses afterward to boost absorption
7. Can repeat 2-3 times daily

Pain Relief for Children and Elderly

Essential oil remedies can provide gentle relief for those with increased pain sensitivity, like children and the elderly. However, certain precautions must be taken:

Children

- Use very diluted oils - 1% or less
- Do not use potentially irritating oils like cinnamon, clove, oregano,
- Opt for soothing, cooling oils like lavender, chamomile,
- Focus more on diffusion than topical applications
- Monitor closely for reactions or sensitivity

Elderly

- Use lower dilutions due to increased skin sensitivity
- Avoid heating pads or compresses to prevent burns
- Monitor closely for skin irritation or sensitivity
- Increase ventilation and avoid overpowering aromas
- Focus on gentle oils like lavender, rose, orange

For the elderly dealing with chronic pain, consistent low-dose aroma exposure via diffusion may offer ongoing comfort and relief without risks of medication side effects. Work closely with doctors for guidance on integrative therapies.

Essential Oils for Headache Relief

Frequent tension headaches plague many adults. Essential oils safely reduce headache pain and nausea through aromatherapeutic inhalation and diluted topical application to the neck, scalp, temples and forehead.

Best oils and methods

- Peppermint, eucalyptus - cooling sensation distracts from pain
- Lavender, rose, and chamomile - relax muscle tension causing headaches
- Clary sage, marjoram - antispasmodic action reduces cramping
- Apply diluted oils to the neck, temple pressure points, and behind the ears
- Inhale oils directly or diffuse them in a room
- Use rollerball applicators for easy topical headache relief

Those prone to headaches can keep essential oil blends on hand for fast-acting, gentle relief of tension headache pain and symptoms without medications.

Natural Anti-Inflammatory Essential Oils

Essential oils like chamomile, helichrysum, lavender and frankincense contain potent anti-inflammatory compounds that help relieve swollen, inflamed, painful tissues when applied topically or inhaled:

- Chamomile - contains chamazulene, bisabolol, matricin, and other anti-inflammatories
- Helichrysum - Flavonoids reduce inflammation, tissue swelling, edema
- Lavender - Linalool linalyl acetate curbs inflammatory prostaglandins
- Frankincense - Boswellic acids powerfully quell inflammation pathways
- Eucalyptus - Antioxidant and analgesic actions reduce inflammatory pain
- Rosemary - Carnosol, carnosic acid, and rosmarinic acid are COX inhibitors
- Marjoram - Terpinenes lower prostaglandin production, causing pain

These and other anti-inflammatory essential oils offer plant-based relief of inflamed muscles, joints, nerves and tissues affected by injury, arthritis or chronic conditions.

Essential Oils for Nerve Pain and Neuropathy

Nerve pain results when nerves are damaged, or inflammation disrupts normal nerve signaling. Gentle essential oils help relieve neuropathic pain when applied topically or diffused:

- Helichrysum – Regenerates nerve tissues, anti-inflammatory, analgesic
- Lavender – Soothes nerve pain, reduces inflammation, restores calm
- Chamomile – Anesthetic, anti-inflammatory, healing properties
- Frankincense – Potent anti-inflammatory, promotes nerve repair
- Rosemary – Analgesic, antioxidant, improves microcirculation
- Eucalyptus – Stimulating properties provide neuropathic pain relief
- Marjoram – Relieves muscle spasms caused by neuropathy

Follow absolute safety protocols and dilute oils very well before applying, starting with low doses. Consistent use can help reset pain signaling disrupted by nerve inflammation and damage over time.

CHAPTER 4

DIGESTIVE HEALTH
(DIGESTIVE AID OILS,
MASSAGE TECHNIQUES)

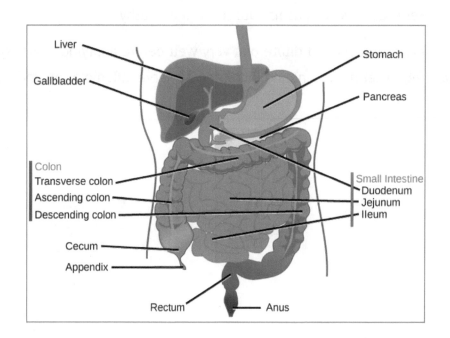

Essential oils can help relieve many types of digestive complaints, including indigestion, nausea, stomach cramps, gas, constipation, diarrhea and food poisoning. Oils contain compounds that directly soothe gastrointestinal tissues, stimulate digestive juices and enzyme secretion, reduce gut spasms and inflammation, inhibit bacterial overgrowth, and calm the enteric nervous system. This chapter explores the most effective digestive aid oils, along with topical massage techniques and aromatherapy recipes, to optimize gut health.

Best Essential Oils for Digestive Problems

Key essential oils to improve various aspects of digestion include:

Peppermint – Smooth muscle relaxant relieves spasms, cramping, gas pain, and nausea. Stimulates bile flow.

Ginger – Warming carminative alleviates nausea, vomiting, gas, diarrhea and stomach cramps.

Lavender – Calms intestinal nervous system overactivity, causing diarrhea, cramping and ulcers.

Chamomile – Anti-inflammatory and antispasmodic eases colic, stomach and bowel inflammation, and gas.

Oregano – Potent antimicrobial activity destroys gut pathogens like Candida, causing indigestion.

Fennel – Carminative, antispasmodic and motility aid effective for gas, cramps, and constipation.

Marjoram – Relieves cramping and soothes nervous indigestion, stomach inflammation and ulcers.

Lemon – Aids digestion encourages digestive enzymes and bile secretion. Disinfects gut.

Black Pepper – Stimulates digestion, bioavailability of nutrients, and peristalsis for constipation.

Using the appropriate oil for each digestive complaint promotes gut health and comfortable digestion.

Topical Abdominal Massage with Essential Oils

Rubbing diluted essential oils over the abdomen area allows active compounds to penetrate and exert local effects on abdominal tissues and organs involved in digestion, including:

- Stomach – Oils like peppermint or lavender relax the stomach and help indigestion.
- Liver – Oils stimulate bile flow detoxification enzymes like lemon rosemary.
- Pancreas – Oils boost digestive enzyme secretion like fennel and cardamom.
- Intestines – Oils reduce gut spasms and inflammation like chamomile marjoram.
- Bladder – Oils support relaxation and microbial balance like sandalwood.

Follow these guidelines for abdominal massage using essential oils:

- Always dilute oils first in a carrier oil like coconut or jojoba oil
- Use light pressure in a clockwise, circular rubbing motion
- Start from the right side under the ribs and work down the intestines
- Follow the path of digestion, focusing on tender, tense areas
- Apply after meals, before bed, during digestive distress
- Use caution over sensitive organs like the liver or kidneys

This direct application method allows essential oils to provide their therapeutic benefits right at the source of digestive discomfort for potent, natural relief of symptoms.

Essential Oil Blends and Recipes for Healthy Digestion

Essential oils can be blended together and incorporated into various remedies and applications to optimize digestion:

Digestive Reliefer Blend:

8 drops peppermint oil 4 drops ginger oil

Five drops of lavender oil Mix with a tablespoon of coconut oil and massage over the abdomen, lower back and feet to aid digestion.

Nausea Relief Rollerball:

8 drops peppermint essential oil, 5 drops ginger essential oil, 7 drops lemon essential oil

10ml rollerball bottle Fill remainder with diluted rubbing alcohol and roll onto wrists and behind ears to curb nausea.

Gas and Bloating Relief Tea:

1 drop fennel essential oil 1 drop lemon essential oil 8 ounces warm chamomile tea Add oils to tea and sip slowly to relieve abdominal bloating, cramping and gas pains.

Bowel Stimulating Bath:

Five drops sweet orange essential oil, 3 drops black pepper essential oil, 1 tablespoon carrier oil. Add to warm bathwater and soak to relieve constipation.

Digestive Vitality Diffuser Blend:

Two drops of ginger essential oil, 3 drops of peppermint essential oil, and 4 drops of coriander essential oil. Diffuse aromatically at mealtimes to invigorate healthy digestion.

Proper use of therapeutic-grade essential oils can alleviate many types of gastrointestinal woes safely and effectively.

Abdominal Massage Directions with Essential Oils

Applying diluted essential oils topically to the abdomen through massage allows direct absorption into the digestive organs to provide symptom relief. Follow these steps:

1. Select 2-3 essential oils appropriate for symptom relief
2. Dilute oils in one tablespoon of carrier oil like coconut or jojoba

3. Rub oil blend lightly over the abdomen in clockwise circles
4. Start from the bottom right quadrant and move up and across
5. Apply extra pressure in areas of pain or tenderness
6. Use lighter pressure over delicate organs like the liver or kidneys
7. Repeat for 5-10 minutes after meals, at bedtime, or when needed

Key tips:

- Never apply undiluted essential oils directly to the skin
- Do not massage directly over swollen organs, tumors, active ulcers
- Seek professional guidance if new abdominal pain develops
- Discontinue use if skin becomes irritated or overly sensitive

Using a healing touch along with aromatherapy allows natural relief of indigestion, gas, constipation and other gastrointestinal issues.

Aromatherapy for Nausea, Vomiting and Upset Stomach

Essential oils known to help relieve nausea, vomiting and upset stomach include:

Peppermint - Settles stomach and reduces nausea through menthol's soothing action on gut muscles and nerves. Also curbs vomiting.

Ginger - Warming and stomach-settling effects combat nausea. Anti-emetic action calms the vomiting reflex.

Lavender - Soothes gastrointestinal smooth muscle spasms, nervous indigestion and vomiting urge center in the brain.

Lemongrass - Alleviates stomach distress and nausea with citral's anti-spasmodic actions.

Chamomile - Gentle anti-inflammatory and antiemetic properties calm the digestive tract.

Fennel - Carminative and motility-regulating effects settle upset digestive tract.

Application tips:

- Inhale oils from cotton balls or diffuse aromatically
- Apply diluted oils behind the ears, on the abdomen, and at the bottom of the feet
- Massage or compress over upset stomach
- Sip fennel, chamomile, ginger or peppermint tea

Rather than suppressing symptoms, essential oils gently relieve causes of nausea like inflammation, spasms, slow digestion and nervous system imbalance for lasting relief.

Essential Oils for Bloating and Abdominal Gas

Abdominal bloating, flatulence and belching can be quite uncomfortable. Essential oils help reduce gas and bloating through their carminative, antispasmodic and stomach-soothing effects when applied topically or inhaled:

Peppermint - Relieves gas pains and pressure. Calms gut muscular contractions, causing cramps.

Chamomile - Soothes inflamed intestinal lining while relaxing smooth muscle spasms causing gas.

Ginger - Acts as a carminative to alleviate gas while easing nausea, spasms, and stomach upset.

Fennel - Antispasmodic digestive aid that relaxes the gut wall while easing flatulence.

Cardamom - Stomach settler that stimulates digestion and helps the body expel gas.

Dill - Digestive stimulant and carminative that relaxes stomach muscles to release gas.

Cumin - Aids digestion and alleviates gassiness through potent carminative actions.

Oils can be diluted in a carrier and then rubbed clockwise over the abdomen to maximize local effects on intestinal tissues. Try a tea with digestive oils like fennel, cardamom or chamomile.

Constipation Relief with Essential Oils

Constipation results from slow gut motility and dehydration. Essential oils increase healthy bowel movements through the following:

- Stimulating peristalsis and digestion
- Soothing gut lining inflammation
- Relaxing clenched pelvic and abdominal muscles
- Encouraging water reabsorption in intestines

Oils that help relieve constipation:

- Sweet orange – Motility stimulant, anti-inflammatory
- Fennel – Carminative, antispasmodic, prokinetic
- Ginger – Warming digestant and gut stimulant
- Black pepper – Stimulates digestive enzymes and motility
- Lavender – Calms muscle spasms and discomfort

- Chamomile – Anti-inflammatory intestinal soother

Drinking tea with digestive oils or diluting in a carrier and massaging over the abdomen and along colon pathways helps bowel movements regulate naturally. Stay well hydrated when using oils to relieve constipation.

Essential Oils for Diarrhea Relief

Diarrhea results from infection, inflammation or nervous system imbalance disrupting normal intestinal fluid reabsorption. Essential oils help control diarrhea through:

- Reducing gut spasms and calming motility
- Soothing intestinal lining irritation
- Slowing hypersensitivity reactions
- Inhibiting microbial growth
- Absorbing toxins released by pathogens

Key anti-diarrheal oils:

- Cinnamon – Inhibits microbial growth, absorbs toxins
- Thyme – Antimicrobial, antispasmodic intestinal effects
- Oregano – Powerful bactericidal and gut-calming actions
- Clove – Antimicrobial, reduces gut hypermotility
- Eucalyptus – Adstringent effect tightens leaky gut
- Ginger – Stomach settling, anti-inflammatory, carminative

Consume essential oils well diluted in cool tea or water to control diarrhea episodes by reducing causative gut inflammation and irritation, calming spasms and inhibiting pathogens.

Aromatherapy for Food Poisoning

Food poisoning causes acute gastrointestinal distress, nausea, diarrhea and dehydration. Essential oils can relieve symptoms and fight pathogens when used aromatically or topically:

- Fennel - Settles the stomach and inhibits gut spasms, causing diarrhea.
- Ginger - Anti-emetic and stomach-soothing actions curb nausea and vomiting.
- Oregano - Potent broad-spectrum antimicrobial properties fight foodborne pathogens.
- Thyme - Antibacterial, antifungal, and antispasmodic intestinal effects.
- Cinnamon - Controls diarrhea while acting as a potent antibacterial agent.

- Peppermint - Relieves stomach and intestinal cramping, nausea and vomiting urge.

Drink very diluted hot tea with cinnamon or oregano oil to combat infection internally. Apply oils like ginger or fennel diluted well with a carrier oil over the abdomen. Diffusing refreshing, antimicrobial oils like lemon or thyme purify the air during recovery.

BOOK 3

ESSENTIAL OILS FOR MENTAL AND EMOTIONAL WELL-BEING

STRESS MANAGEMENT AND RELAXATION

(CALMING OILS, DIFFUSION METHODS)

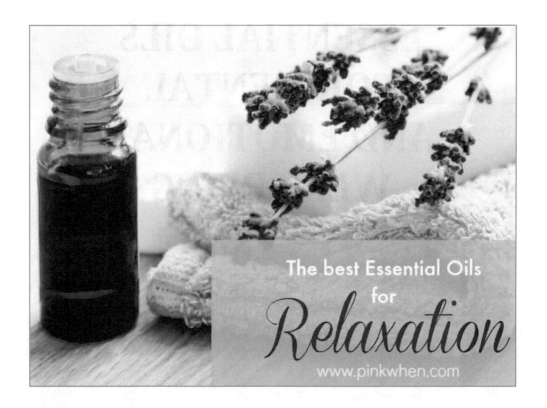

In today's fast-paced world, stress has become a ubiquitous and often overwhelming part of our lives. Balancing the demands of work, relationships, and personal responsibilities can leave us mentally and emotionally drained. The pursuit of relaxation and effective stress management has driven many individuals to explore natural remedies, and among the most promising options are essential oils. These precious plant extracts have been used for centuries for their therapeutic properties, particularly in promoting relaxation and tranquility.

Understanding Stress and Its Impact

Before delving into the world of essential oils and how they can aid in stress management, it's essential to understand what stress is and how it affects us. Stress is the body's natural response to perceived threats or challenges. When we encounter a stressful situation, our bodies release hormones like adrenaline and cortisol, which prepare us for the "fight or flight" response. This response can be beneficial in the short term, but chronic stress can have detrimental effects on our physical and mental health.

Prolonged stress can lead to a range of health problems, including anxiety, depression, cardiovascular issues, and weakened immune function. Additionally, stress can disrupt our sleep patterns, impair our ability to concentrate, and negatively impact our relationships. It's clear that finding effective ways to manage and alleviate stress is essential for our overall well-being.

Popular Calming Essential Oils

Several essential oils are renowned for their stress-relieving properties. Let's explore some of the most popular ones:

Lavender (Lavandula angustifolia)

Perhaps the most famous of all calming essential oils, lavender has a gentle, floral aroma that is instantly recognizable. Lavender oil is known for its ability to soothe the nervous system, making it an excellent choice for reducing anxiety and promoting relaxation. It's often used to facilitate better sleep and combat insomnia.

Chamomile (Matricaria chamomilla)

Chamomile essential oil, with its mild and comforting scent, is another effective option for reducing stress and promoting relaxation. It has anti-anxiety properties and is often used in aromatherapy to create a sense of calm and tranquility.

Bergamot (Citrus bergamia)

Bergamot essential oil has a citrusy and uplifting aroma. While it is known for its mood-enhancing properties, it's also effective in reducing anxiety and tension. Bergamot is often used to alleviate symptoms of depression and stress-related disorders.

Frankincense (Boswellia carterii)

Frankincense essential oil is revered for its grounding and spiritually uplifting qualities. It can help reduce stress and anxiety by promoting deep relaxation and enhancing feelings of inner peace and contentment.

Effective Diffusion Methods

Now that we have explored some of the calming essential oils let's dive into the various diffusion methods that allow us to harness their power for stress management.

Ultrasonic Diffusers

Ultrasonic diffusers are among the most popular choices for diffusing essential oils. These devices use ultrasonic vibrations to break down essential oils and water into fine mist particles, dispersing them into the air. Ultrasonic diffusers are known for their quiet operation and the ability to maintain the therapeutic properties of essential oils.

Nebulizing Diffusers

Nebulizing diffusers work by using pressurized air to atomize essential oils into tiny particles that are released into the air. They do not require water or heat, which means that the oil's chemical composition remains intact. Nebulizing diffusers are excellent for delivering a concentrated burst of essential oil aroma, making them ideal for larger spaces.

Evaporative Diffusers

Evaporative diffusers use a fan or a gentle stream of air to evaporate essential oils from a pad or surface. As the oils evaporate, they disperse into the surrounding air. While these diffusers are simple and affordable, they may not be as effective in maintaining the therapeutic properties of essential oils as ultrasonic or nebulizing diffusers.

Heat Diffusers

Heat diffusers, such as candle diffusers and electric heat diffusers, use heat to evaporate essential oils. While they can be effective in releasing the aroma of essential oils, they may alter the chemical composition of the oils, potentially reducing their therapeutic benefits.

Personal Inhalers

Personal inhalers are compact and portable devices that allow you to inhale the aroma of essential oils directly. These are particularly useful for on-the-go stress relief. You can add a few drops of calming essential oil to a wick or cotton pad inside the inhaler and inhale deeply whenever you need a moment of relaxation.

The Science Behind Aromatherapy and Stress Reduction

Aromatherapy, the practice of using essential oils for therapeutic purposes, is based on the idea that the aromatic compounds in these oils can influence our mood, emotions, and overall well-being. While aromatherapy has been used for centuries, modern scientific research has provided insights into how essential oils interact with our bodies to reduce stress and induce relaxation.

The Olfactory System

When we inhale the aroma of essential oils, it triggers our olfactory system, which is responsible for our sense of smell. The olfactory system is intricately connected to the limbic system, the part of the brain that regulates emotions and memories. This connection allows the aroma of essential oils to directly impact our emotional state.

Chemical Compounds

Essential oils are complex mixtures of chemical compounds, and each oil contains a unique combination of these compounds. Some compounds found in calming essential oils, such as linalool in lavender and chamomile, have been shown to have relaxing and sedative effects. Others, like limonene in bergamot, can enhance mood and reduce anxiety.

Clinical Studies

Numerous clinical studies have explored the effects of specific essential oils on stress and anxiety. For example, a study published in the journal "Complementary Therapies in Clinical Practice" in 2016 found that inhaling a blend of lavender, bergamot, and frankincense essential oils reduced anxiety and improved sleep quality in patients with generalized anxiety disorder.

CHAPTER 2

MOOD ENHANCEMENT
(UPLIFTING OILS, AROMATHERAPY BLENDS)

Our emotions have a profound impact on our overall well-being. At times, life's challenges, stressors, or simply the daily grind can leave us feeling down, anxious, or overwhelmed. Fortunately, nature provides us with a beautiful remedy in the form of essential oils. These aromatic compounds extracted from various plants have the power to influence our mood positively and uplift our spirits, making them invaluable tools for promoting mental and emotional wellness.

In this chapter, we will explore the world of uplifting essential oils, delve into their fascinating properties, and dive deep into the art of aromatherapy blends. We will discover how these oils can be harnessed to enhance our mood and create customized blends that cater to our individual preferences and needs.

The Science Behind Mood Enhancement

Before we embark on our journey into the world of uplifting essential oils and aromatherapy blends, it's essential to understand the science behind how these aromatic compounds interact with our brains and bodies to influence our mood.

Olfactory System

The olfactory system, responsible for our sense of smell, plays a pivotal role in how essential oils impact our emotions. When we inhale the aroma of an essential oil, odor molecules stimulate receptors in the nasal cavity, sending signals to the brain's limbic system. This part of the brain is responsible for emotions, memory, and mood regulation, making it the epicenter of essential oil-induced mood enhancement.

Chemical Composition

Each essential oil contains a unique chemical composition that determines its therapeutic properties. For mood enhancement, we focus on oils rich in specific compounds. For instance, citrus oils like lemon and orange are high in limonene and are known for their mood-lifting and stress-reducing effects. The terpene linalool, found in lavender and other calming oils, is known for its anxiety-reducing properties.

Absorption

Essential oils can be absorbed through the skin, particularly when diluted and applied topically. They can also be absorbed through inhalation, where the aromatic molecules enter the bloodstream via the lungs. This dual absorption method allows for versatility in how we use essential oils for mood enhancement.

Uplifting Essential Oils

Now that we have a foundational understanding of how essential oils interact with our bodies let's explore some of the most effective and popular uplifting essential oils.

Citrus Oils

- Lemon: Known for its bright, zesty scent, lemon oil is a natural mood enhancer. It can help alleviate stress, boost energy levels, and create a sense of positivity.
- Sweet Orange: With its sweet and fruity aroma, sweet orange oil is a powerful mood lifter. It can help reduce anxiety and promote a cheerful disposition.
- Grapefruit: This refreshing oil has a balancing effect on emotions. It can reduce mental fatigue and uplift the spirit.

Peppermint

Peppermint oil's invigorating scent is ideal for boosting focus and alertness. It can help combat mental fatigue and create a sense of clarity.

Eucalyptus

Eucalyptus oil's fresh and camphoraceous aroma is excellent for providing mental clarity and promoting a feeling of refreshment.

Bergamot

Bergamot oil, derived from the bergamot orange, has a unique citrusy-floral scent. It is known for its mood-enhancing and anxiety-reducing properties.

Ylang-Ylang

Ylang-ylang oil boasts a sweet and floral fragrance that can soothe the nervous system and promote feelings of joy and relaxation.

Creating Aromatherapy Blends for Mood Enhancement

One of the most exciting aspects of using essential oils for mood enhancement is the art of crafting aromatherapy blends. Blending allows us to combine different essential oils to create unique and personalized scents that cater to our specific emotional needs and preferences. Below, we will explore the steps to creating your aromatherapy blends.

Step 1: Choose Your Base Oils

Base oils, also known as carrier oils, serve as the foundation for your aromatherapy blend. They dilute the potent essential oils, making them safe for topical application and helping to disperse the aroma. Common carrier oils include jojoba oil, sweet almond oil, and fractionated coconut oil. Consider your skin type and any allergies when selecting a carrier oil.

Step 2: Select Your Uplifting Essential Oils

Once you've chosen your base oil, it's time to select the uplifting essential oils that will form the heart of your blend. Start by considering the specific mood you want to enhance. Do you need a blend of energy and positivity, or perhaps one for relaxation and stress relief? Here are a few example blends:

Energizing Blend:

To boost your energy and motivation, combine sweet orange, lemon, and peppermint essential oils in a carrier oil. This blend can be applied to pulse points or used in a roller bottle for easy application throughout the day.

Relaxation Blend:

For moments of calm and relaxation, mix lavender, ylang-ylang, and bergamot essential oils in a carrier oil. This blend is perfect for a soothing massage or added to a warm bath.

Step 3: Determine the Dilution Ratio

The dilution ratio refers to the proportion of essential oil to carrier oil in your blend. This ratio is crucial because it ensures that the essential oils are properly diluted to avoid skin irritation. A common dilution ratio for adults is 2-3% essential oil to carrier oil. For example, if you're making a 10 ml roller bottle, you would add 6-9 drops of essential oil to the carrier oil.

Step 4: Blend and Test

Carefully combine the chosen essential oils with your carrier oil in a glass container. Use a glass dropper to measure the essential oils accurately. Once blended, it's a good practice to perform a skin patch test to ensure there are no adverse reactions. Apply a small amount of the blend to your forearm and wait 24 hours to check for any redness, itching, or irritation.

Step 5: Store and Enjoy

Once you've created your aromatherapy blend, store it in a dark glass bottle to protect it from light and air, which can degrade the essential oils. Label your blend with the date and ingredients for future reference. Use your custom blend as needed to enhance your mood, either by applying it to your skin, diffusing it, or adding it to a warm bath.

Practical Applications of Aromatherapy Blends

Aromatherapy blends can be used in various ways to enhance your mood and promote emotional well-being. Here are some practical applications:

1. Personal Inhalers: You can create portable inhalers filled with your mood-enhancing blends. Inhaling the aroma throughout the day can help maintain a positive mindset.
2. Diffusion: Use an essential oil diffuser to disperse the uplifting scent throughout your home or workspace. This is particularly effective when you need to create a conducive environment for work or relaxation.
3. Massage and Body Oils: Diluted aromatherapy blends make excellent massage oils. A soothing massage can not only relax your muscles but also lift your spirits.
4. Bath Additives: Enhance your bath time by adding a few drops of your custom blend to warm bathwater. The soothing scent can help you unwind and de-stress.
5. Perfume: Create a natural, personalized perfume by applying your blend to pulse points, such as wrists and neck.

Uplifting essential oils and the art of aromatherapy blending provide us with a delightful and effective means to positively influence our mood and emotional state. By understanding the science behind these oils and learning how to craft personalized aromatherapy blends, we can take charge of our well-being and infuse our lives with moments of joy, relaxation, and clarity. Explore the vast array of essential oils and let your creativity guide you as you discover the transformative power of aromatherapy for mood enhancement and emotional balance.

CHAPTER 3

FOCUS AND CONCENTRATION

(STIMULATING OILS, INHALATION TECHNIQUES)

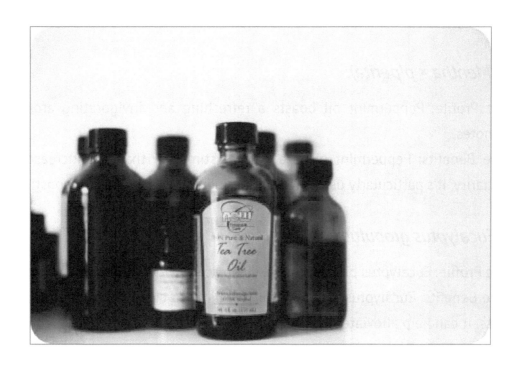

I n today's fast-paced and information-driven world, maintaining focus and concentration is a constant challenge. Whether you're a student trying to excel in academics, a professional striving to meet tight deadlines, or simply seeking improved productivity, the ability to stay focused and attentive is paramount. Distractions are everywhere, vying for our attention, and often, we find ourselves struggling to stay on task. This chapter delves into the world of stimulating essential oils and explores various effective inhalation techniques that can help sharpen focus, enhance cognitive function, and promote a clear state of mind.

Understanding Stimulating Essential Oils

Essential oils are potent plant extracts renowned for their therapeutic properties. When it comes to improving focus and concentration, certain essential oils stand out due to their stimulating and invigorating qualities. These oils work by stimulating the brain and promoting mental clarity, making it easier to concentrate on tasks at hand. Here are some of the key stimulating essential oils:

Rosemary (Rosmarinus officinalis):

- Aromatic Profile: Rosemary oil has a fresh, herbaceous scent with hints of camphor and woodiness.
- Cognitive Benefits: Rosemary is known to enhance memory retention and alertness. It can help improve concentration and cognitive function, making it an ideal choice for tasks that require mental acuity.

Peppermint (Mentha × piperita):

- Aromatic Profile: Peppermint oil boasts a refreshing and invigorating aroma with minty, cooling notes.
- Cognitive Benefits: Peppermint oil is a natural stimulant that can increase alertness and mental clarity. It's particularly useful for combating mental fatigue and boosting focus.

Eucalyptus (Eucalyptus globulus):

- Aromatic Profile: Eucalyptus oil has a fresh, clean scent with a hint of camphor and earthiness.
- Cognitive Benefits: Eucalyptus is known for its ability to clear the mind and promote mental sharpness. It can help alleviate mental exhaustion and promote focus.

Lemon (Citrus limon):

- Aromatic Profile: Lemon oil offers a bright and uplifting citrus scent.
- Cognitive Benefits: Lemon oil is excellent for improving mood and concentration. It can uplift spirits and enhance cognitive performance.

Basil (Ocimum basilicum):

- Aromatic Profile: Basil oil has a warm, spicy-sweet aroma with herbal undertones.
- Cognitive Benefits: Basil is believed to enhance mental alertness and concentration. It can provide mental clarity and support overall cognitive function.

Effective Inhalation Techniques

Now that we've explored the stimulating essential oils that can enhance focus and concentration let's delve into the various inhalation techniques that can help you make the most of these aromatic wonders.

Direct Inhalation

Direct inhalation is one of the simplest and most immediate ways to experience the benefits of stimulating essential oils. It involves inhaling the aroma of the oil directly from the bottle or a few drops applied to a tissue or cotton ball. Here's how to do it:

1. Choose the stimulating essential oil of your preference.
2. Uncap the bottle and hold it about an inch away from your nose.
3. Take a deep breath through your nose, inhaling the aroma deeply.
4. Exhale slowly and repeat the process as needed.

This technique is ideal for quick bursts of focus and concentration. It's portable and can be used virtually anywhere, whether you're at work, studying, or in need of a mental pick-me-up.

Personal Inhalers

Personal inhalers are convenient devices designed for essential oil inhalation. They consist of a small tube or container with a wick or absorbent pad inside. Here's how to use a personal inhaler for focus and concentration:

1. Select your desired stimulating essential oil or a blend.
2. Apply a few drops of the oil onto the absorbent pad inside the inhaler.
3. Insert the pad into the tube and seal it.
4. Whenever you need a concentration boost, remove the cap and inhale deeply through the inhaler.

Personal inhalers are discrete and can be carried in your pocket or purse, making them an excellent option for on-the-go focus support.

Diffusion

Diffusion involves using an essential oil diffuser to disperse the aroma of stimulating oils into the air. This method creates a continuous stream of the oil's scent in your environment, promoting an ongoing sense of alertness and focus. Here's how to use a diffuser for cognitive enhancement:

1. Fill your diffuser with water according to the manufacturer's instructions.
2. Add a few drops (typically 3-5 drops) of your chosen stimulating essential oil.
3. Turn on the diffuser and let it run for the recommended duration.

Diffusers come in various types, including ultrasonic, nebulizing, and evaporative diffusers, each offering its own unique benefits. Ultrasonic diffusers use water to disperse the oils into a fine mist while nebulizing diffusers break the oils into tiny particles without water. Both methods are effective in delivering the aromatic benefits of essential oils.

Steam Inhalation

Steam inhalation is an age-old technique that can be used to enhance focus and clear the mind. It involves adding stimulating essential oils to a bowl of hot water and inhaling the steam. Here's how to do it:

1. Boil a pot of water and transfer it to a heatproof bowl.
2. Add a few drops of your chosen stimulating essential oil to the hot water.
3. Place your face a safe distance above the bowl, covering your head with a towel to trap the steam.
4. Close your eyes and inhale deeply through your nose.

Steam inhalation not only supports focus but can also alleviate sinus congestion and respiratory issues.

Topical Application

While inhalation is the primary method for stimulating essential oils, topical application can also be effective. Applying diluted essential oils to specific pulse points or using them in massage oils can promote mental clarity and alertness. However, it's important to dilute essential oils properly with a carrier oil to avoid skin irritation.

1. Choose a carrier oil such as jojoba, almond, or coconut oil.
2. Mix a few drops of the stimulating essential oil with the carrier oil (typically a 2-3% dilution).
3. Apply the blend to your temples, wrists, or the back of your neck.
4. Gently massage the oil into your skin.

This method not only delivers the benefits of the oil through your skin but also engages your sense of touch, providing an additional sensory experience.

Yoga and Meditation

Yoga and meditation practices often incorporate essential oils to enhance the mind-body connection and promote focus. A few drops of stimulating essential oils can be added to a diffuser or applied to pulse points before beginning your practice. The combination of aromatherapy and mindful movement or meditation can be especially effective in achieving mental clarity and concentration.

DIY Blends for Focus and Concentration

Crafting your own essential oil blends tailored to your specific needs can be a rewarding experience. Here's a simple DIY recipe for a focus-enhancing blend:

Ingredients:

- 10 drops of Rosemary essential oil
- 8 drops Peppermint essential oil
- 7 drops Lemon essential oil
- 5 drops of Basil essential oil
- 1 oz (30 ml) carrier oil (e.g., jojoba, sweet almond)

Directions:

1. In an amber glass bottle, add the essential oils.
2. Top up the bottle with the carrier oil and seal it.
3. Gently shake the bottle to mix the oils.
4. Apply this blend to your pulse points or use it in a personal inhaler for a potent focus-enhancing experience.

CHAPTER 4

SLEEP SUPPORT

(SOOTHING OILS, BEDTIME RITUALS)

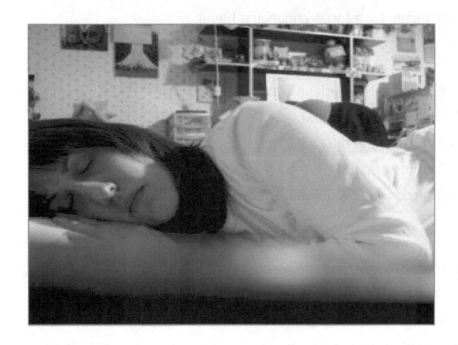

I n our busy lives, achieving a restful and rejuvenating night's sleep can sometimes feel elusive. The demands of work, family, and other responsibilities can leave us restless and stressed, making it challenging to unwind and fall asleep easily. This chapter explores the realm of soothing essential oils and bedtime rituals, offering a natural and effective approach to enhancing the quality of our sleep.

Understanding the Sleep Cycle

Before delving into the solutions that soothing essential oils and bedtime rituals offer, it's crucial to understand the sleep cycle. Sleep is divided into several stages, including non-rapid eye movement (NREM) stages and rapid eye movement (REM) stages. NREM stages progress from light to deep sleep, while REM sleep is when most dreaming occurs. A complete sleep cycle typically lasts around 90 to 110 minutes, and ideally, one should experience multiple cycles throughout the night.

Soothing Essential Oils for Sleep Support

Lavender Oil

Lavender oil is a star player in the realm of essential oils for promoting sleep and relaxation. Its gentle, floral aroma is known for its calming and soothing effects on the nervous system. Lavender oil helps reduce anxiety, lower blood pressure, and induce a sense of tranquility, making it an excellent choice for those seeking a peaceful night's sleep.

Using Lavender Oil for Sleep:

a. Diffusion: Add a few drops of lavender oil to a diffuser and let the aromatic mist fill your bedroom before bedtime.

b. Pillow Spray: Mix a few drops of lavender oil with water in a spray bottle and lightly mist your pillow and bedding.

c. Bath: Incorporate a few drops of lavender oil into a warm bath before bedtime for a relaxing pre-sleep soak.

Roman Chamomile Oil

Roman chamomile oil, derived from the chamomile flower, is renowned for its gentle and calming properties. It's often used to reduce stress, anxiety, and restlessness, helping to create a serene atmosphere conducive to restful sleep.

Using Roman Chamomile Oil for Sleep:

a. Massage: Dilute Roman chamomile oil with a carrier oil like sweet almond or jojoba oil and massage it into the skin before bedtime.

b. Inhalation: Add a few drops to a bowl of hot water, cover your head with a towel, and inhale the steam for a calming experience.

c. Diffusion: Diffuse Roman chamomile oil in your bedroom using a diffuser to infuse the air with its soothing aroma.

Cedarwood Oil

Cedarwood oil, obtained from cedarwood trees, possesses a warm, woody scent that promotes relaxation and tranquility. It's known to have sedative effects, making it an excellent choice for those struggling with insomnia or restless sleep.

Using Cedarwood Oil for Sleep:

a. Diffusion: Add a few drops of cedarwood oil to a diffuser in your bedroom to create a calming ambiance.

b. Topical Application: Dilute cedarwood oil with a carrier oil and apply it to the bottoms of your feet or your wrists before bedtime.

c. Bedding Spray: Create a natural bedding spray by mixing cedarwood oil with water and spritzing it lightly on your pillows and sheets.

BOOK 4

ESSENTIAL OILS FOR SKINCARE AND BEAUTY

CHAPTER 1

FACIAL CARE
(CLEANSING, TONING, MOISTURIZING)

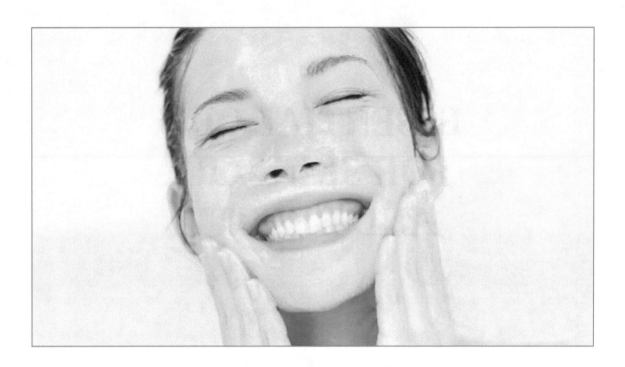

Facial care is the cornerstone of any effective skincare routine. It is a daily ritual that helps maintain the health and radiance of your skin. In this chapter, we will explore the world of facial care, focusing on the three essential steps: cleansing, toning, and moisturizing. We will delve into the science behind these practices and the remarkable role that essential oils play in enhancing the efficacy of these skincare rituals.

Cleansing with Essential Oils

Cleansing is the fundamental step in any skincare routine. It is the process of removing impurities, dirt, excess oil, and makeup from the skin's surface. A proper cleansing routine ensures that your skin is a clean canvas, ready to absorb the benefits of the subsequent skincare products.

The Role of Essential Oils in Cleansing

Essential oils offer a natural and effective way to cleanse the skin. Many essential oils, such as lavender, tea tree, and chamomile, possess antibacterial, antimicrobial, and anti-inflammatory properties. These properties make them excellent choices for gentle yet thorough cleansing.

Lavender Oil

Lavender oil is well-known for its soothing and calming properties. When used in a cleanser, it not only helps remove impurities but also provides a sense of relaxation during your skincare routine. Additionally, lavender oil has antimicrobial properties, making it beneficial for those with acne-prone skin.

Tea Tree Oil

Tea tree oil is a powerful natural antiseptic. It can effectively cleanse the skin, especially for those with oily and acne-prone skin. Tea tree oil helps reduce inflammation and fights acne-causing bacteria, making it an essential ingredient in many cleansers.

Chamomile Oil

Chamomile oil is gentle and suitable for sensitive skin. It has anti-inflammatory and soothing properties, making it an ideal choice for cleansing delicate facial skin. Chamomile oil can help reduce redness and irritation while cleansing.

How to Cleanse with Essential Oils

To cleanse your face effectively with essential oils, follow these steps:

1. Look for a cleanser that contains essential oils suitable for your skin type. For example, if you have oily skin, opt for a cleanser with tea tree oil. If you have sensitive skin, choose one with chamomile oil.
2. If you're wearing makeup, consider using a gentle makeup remover or oil-based cleanser to dissolve makeup before using your essential oil-based cleanser.
3. Wet your face with lukewarm water and apply the cleanser with gentle, upward circular motions. Be sure to avoid the eye area unless your cleanser is specifically designed for that purpose.
4. Rinse your face with lukewarm water until all traces of the cleanser are removed. Pat your face dry with a clean towel.

Toning with Essential Oils

Toning is the second step in facial care. It involves using a toner or a toning product to balance the skin's pH levels, tighten pores, and prepare the skin for the next steps in your skincare routine.

The Role of Essential Oils in Toning

Essential oils such as rosemary, witch hazel, and frankincense are renowned for their astringent properties, making them excellent choices for toning the skin.

Rosemary Oil

Rosemary oil is known for its astringent properties, which help tighten and tone the skin. It also has antioxidant properties that can protect the skin from free radical damage.

Witch Hazel

Witch hazel is a natural astringent and anti-inflammatory agent. It helps reduce the size of pores, control excess oil, and soothe irritated skin.

Frankincense Oil

Frankincense oil is not only astringent but also has skin-regenerating properties. It can help improve skin elasticity and reduce the appearance of fine lines and wrinkles.

How to Tone with Essential Oils

To tone your face effectively with essential oils, follow these steps:

1. Look for a toner that contains essential oils suitable for your skin type. Rosemary, witch hazel, and frankincense are great choices for various skin types.
2. After cleansing, apply the toner to a cotton pad and gently swipe it across your face, avoiding the eye area.
3. Let the toner absorb into your skin for a minute or two before moving on to the next step in your skincare routine.

Moisturizing with Essential Oils

Moisturizing is the final step in facial care. It involves applying a moisturizer or moisturizing product to hydrate the skin and lock in moisture. Proper moisturization is essential for maintaining skin hydration, suppleness, and a healthy barrier.

The Role of Essential Oils in Moisturizing

Certain essential oils, such as jojoba, rosehip, and geranium, are excellent choices for moisturizing the skin. These oils are well-tolerated by most skin types and offer numerous benefits beyond hydration.

Jojoba Oil

Jojoba oil is known for its similarity to the skin's natural sebum, making it an ideal moisturizer for all skin types. It is lightweight and easily absorbed, providing long-lasting hydration without clogging pores.

Rosehip Oil

Rosehip oil is rich in vitamins A and C, as well as essential fatty acids. It not only moisturizes the skin but also helps improve skin elasticity, reduce the signs of aging, and fade scars and hyperpigmentation.

Geranium Oil

Geranium oil has a balancing effect on the skin, making it suitable for both oily and dry skin types. It can help regulate oil production while providing hydration and a pleasant fragrance.

How to Moisturize with Essential Oils

To moisturize your face effectively with essential oils, follow these steps:

1. Look for a moisturizer that contains essential oils suitable for your skin type. Jojoba, rosehip, and geranium oils are commonly found in moisturizing products.
2. After toning, apply a small amount of moisturizer to your face and neck using gentle upward strokes. Massage the moisturizer into your skin to ensure even coverage.
3. Give the moisturizer a few minutes to absorb into your skin before applying any makeup or moving on to other skincare steps.

Facial care is an essential aspect of maintaining healthy, glowing skin. The three fundamental steps of facial care—cleansing, toning, and moisturizing—are crucial for a successful skincare routine.

CHAPTER 2

BODY CARE
(EXFOLIATION, HYDRATION, CELLULITE TREATMENT)

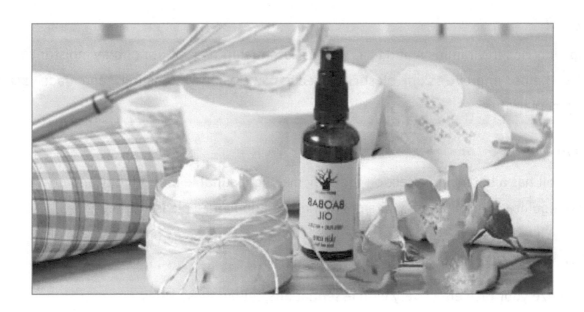

In the realm of skincare and beauty, our bodies deserve just as much attention as our faces. The health and appearance of our skin across our entire body contribute significantly to our overall self-confidence and well-being. This chapter focuses on body care, emphasizing the use of essential oils for exfoliation, hydration, and cellulite treatment—a comprehensive approach to nurturing and beautifying our bodies.

Exfoliation with Essential Oils

Exfoliation is a crucial step in maintaining healthy and glowing skin. It involves the removal of dead skin cells from the surface, allowing new cells to regenerate and revealing a smoother, more radiant complexion. While there are various methods of exfoliation, incorporating essential oils into this process can significantly enhance its efficacy and overall experience.

When seeking to exfoliate the body, essential oils can serve as natural exfoliants, providing a gentle yet effective way to slough off dead skin cells. The utilization of essential oils for this purpose is rooted in their inherent properties, including anti-inflammatory, antiseptic, and aromatic characteristics.

Properties of Essential Oils for Exfoliation

Essential oils derived from plants, flowers, and fruits offer diverse properties that make them ideal for exfoliation. For instance, citrus essential oils such as lemon and grapefruit possess astringent qualities that help tighten the skin and reduce excess oil. Peppermint oil is invigorating and can stimulate blood circulation, aiding in a revitalizing exfoliation experience. Lavender oil, on the other hand, is gentle and calming, making it suitable for sensitive skin types.

Exfoliation Techniques with Essential Oils

The versatility of essential oils allows for a variety of exfoliation techniques. One popular method is creating a DIY exfoliating scrub by combining essential oils with natural exfoliants like sugar, salt, or coffee grounds. The essential oils act as not only aromatic enhancers but also skin-rejuvenating agents.

To make an exfoliating scrub, simply mix the chosen exfoliant with a carrier oil (such as coconut or jojoba oil) and a few drops of the selected essential oil(s). This concoction can then be gently massaged onto damp skin, effectively removing dead skin cells and leaving the skin feeling soft and revitalized.

Benefits of Essential Oil Exfoliation

Beyond removing dead skin cells, essential oil exfoliation offers additional benefits. The massage action during exfoliation helps stimulate blood circulation, which can contribute to improved skin texture and even tone. Moreover, essential oils infuse the skin with their therapeutic properties, providing a sense of relaxation and promoting overall skin health.

Regular exfoliation with essential oils can enhance the absorption of subsequent skincare products, allowing moisturizers and serums to penetrate deeper into the skin for optimal effectiveness. This ensures that the skin receives the maximum benefits of the applied products.

Hydration with Essential Oils

Skin hydration is a cornerstone of good skincare, promoting a supple and youthful complexion. Adequate hydration helps maintain the skin's natural moisture balance, preventing dryness, flakiness, and discomfort. Essential oils, with their emollient and hydrating properties, can play a significant role in ensuring the skin stays moisturized and nourished.

Hydrating Properties of Essential Oils

Essential oils are known for their ability to lock in moisture and prevent water loss from the skin. Oils such as coconut, sweet almond, and avocado are rich in fatty acids that deeply hydrate and replenish the skin's moisture levels. These oils provide a protective barrier, keeping the skin soft and hydrated throughout the day.

Incorporating Essential Oils into a Hydration Routine

Including essential oils in a daily hydration routine is simple and effective. These oils can be used directly on the skin or mixed with a preferred carrier oil or moisturizer. Applying a few drops of essential oil-infused carrier oil after a shower or bath helps seal in moisture, leaving the skin feeling soft and supple.

Additionally, essential oils can be infused into mists or toners, providing a quick and refreshing burst of hydration throughout the day. A spritz of water and essential oil blend can rejuvenate the skin, making it an ideal addition to a skincare routine, especially in dry or arid climates.

Benefits of Hydrating with Essential Oils

Hydrating with essential oils offers numerous benefits beyond moisturizing the skin. These oils often contain vitamins, antioxidants, and other nutrients that support overall skin health. The hydrating process helps maintain the skin's elasticity, reducing the appearance of fine lines and wrinkles and promoting a youthful complexion.

Essential oils also possess aromatherapeutic properties that can enhance relaxation and reduce stress. The application of these oils in a hydrating routine offers the dual benefit of nurturing both the skin and the mind, creating a holistic and rejuvenating experience.

Cellulite Treatment with Essential Oils

Cellulite, characterized by the dimpling of the skin, especially around the thighs and buttocks, is a common concern for many individuals. While cellulite is natural and not harmful, some may wish to minimize its appearance for cosmetic reasons. Essential oils, renowned for their potential in skin rejuvenation and toning, are often explored for their cellulite-reducing properties.

Properties of Essential Oils for Cellulite Treatment

Certain essential oils possess properties that can aid in reducing the appearance of cellulite. For instance, juniper essential oil is known for its detoxifying and diuretic properties, helping to eliminate excess fluids from the body. Grapefruit essential oil is believed to have a stimulating effect on the lymphatic system, assisting in the reduction of cellulite.

Application Techniques for Cellulite Treatment

Utilizing essential oils for cellulite treatment involves targeted massage and application techniques. A popular approach is creating a massage oil blend by diluting essential oils with a carrier oil like coconut or jojoba oil. This blend can then be massaged onto the affected areas using circular motions, aiding in stimulating blood circulation and breaking down fat deposits.

Regular massage with essential oil blends can help improve the skin's texture and reduce the appearance of cellulite over time. It's important to maintain consistency and complement this treatment with a healthy diet and regular exercise for optimal results.

Benefits of Essential Oil Cellulite Treatment

Incorporating essential oils into a cellulite treatment routine offers a natural and non-invasive approach to addressing this concern. The massage process itself, along with the application of essential oils, promotes relaxation and improved blood circulation, contributing to healthier-looking skin.

While essential oils may not provide a permanent solution to cellulite, they can assist in minimizing its appearance and improving skin tone. The aromatherapeutic effects of these oils also contribute to a sense of well-being during the treatment, enhancing the overall experience.

CHAPTER 3

HAIR CARE
(STRENGTHENING, NOURISHING, SCALP HEALTH)

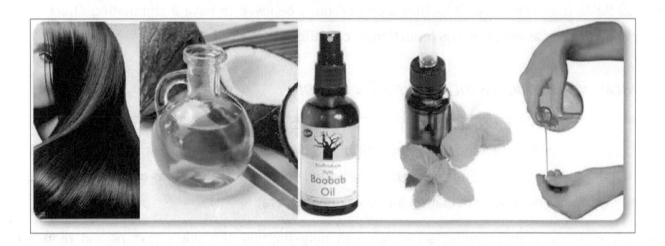

Our hair, a defining aspect of our beauty and identity, requires diligent care to maintain its health, strength, and luster. Hair care encompasses a broad spectrum of practices, from cleansing to styling, and is essential for achieving the desired look and ensuring the longevity of our locks. In this chapter, we will embark on a comprehensive exploration of utilizing essential oils to fortify and nourish our hair while also focusing on maintaining a healthy scalp—a foundation for robust hair growth.

Strengthening Hair with Essential Oils

Hair strength is a fundamental factor that contributes to its overall appearance and resilience against various external stressors. Essential oils, derived from plant sources, offer a natural and effective way to enhance the strength of our hair. Among the numerous essential oils recognized for their hair-strengthening properties, rosemary, lavender, and cedarwood stand out prominently.

Rosemary essential oil, extracted from the Rosmarinus officinalis plant, is celebrated for its remarkable ability to stimulate hair growth and strengthen hair follicles. It increases circulation in the scalp, providing the hair roots with enhanced nourishment and oxygen. This, in turn, promotes thicker and stronger hair strands, reducing hair loss and breakage.

Lavender essential oil, obtained from Lavandula angustifolia flowers, is widely known for its soothing and calming properties. However, it also plays a pivotal role in strengthening hair. Lavender oil nourishes the hair follicles, assisting in preventing hair loss and promoting the growth of new hair. Its gentle nature makes it suitable for those with sensitive scalps.

Cedarwood essential oil, derived from the wood of cedar trees, possesses potent antifungal and antibacterial properties. It helps maintain a healthy scalp by combating conditions like dandruff and infections that may hinder hair growth. Additionally, cedarwood oil regulates oil production in the scalp, contributing to a balanced and nourished environment for the hair to flourish.

To harness the strengthening benefits of these essential oils, a blend can be created by combining a few drops of each oil with a carrier oil such as jojoba or coconut oil. This blend can be gently massaged into the scalp and left on for a designated period before washing. Regular application of this concoction can lead to stronger, more resilient hair and a healthier scalp.

Nourishing Hair with Essential Oils

Nourishment is an essential aspect of hair care, as it directly impacts the texture, shine, and overall health of our locks. Essential oils possess a treasure trove of vitamins, minerals, and fatty acids that provide the hair with the nourishment it needs to thrive. Among the most beneficial essential oils for hair nourishment are argan oil, coconut oil, and jojoba oil.

Argan oil

Argan oil, often referred to as "liquid gold," is derived from the kernels of the Argania spinosa tree, native to Morocco. It is rich in essential fatty acids and vitamin E, which work synergistically to nourish and moisturize the hair, leaving it soft, smooth, and manageable. Argan oil also helps repair damaged hair and reduce frizz, making it a popular choice for hair nourishment.

Coconut oil

Coconut oil, obtained from the meat of coconuts, is a versatile and deeply nourishing oil. It contains lauric acid, which penetrates the hair shaft and provides strength and moisture from within. Coconut oil helps prevent protein loss in hair, making it an effective nourishing treatment for damaged and brittle hair. It also imparts a natural shine and smoothness to the hair.

Jojoba oil

Jojoba oil, extracted from the seeds of the jojoba plant, closely resembles the natural oils produced by the scalp. This makes it an excellent oil for nourishing the hair without leaving it greasy. Jojoba oil helps balance the scalp's oil production, making it suitable for various hair types. It nourishes the hair strands, promoting strength and vitality.

Creating a nourishing hair treatment using essential oils involves blending a few drops of the chosen oils with a carrier oil. This blend can be applied to damp or dry hair, focusing on the ends and working upwards. Leaving it on for a sufficient amount of time allows the oils to penetrate and nourish the hair. Regular use of this treatment can result in softer, more manageable hair that exudes a healthy glow.

Scalp Health with Essential Oils

The foundation of a healthy head of hair lies in a well-nourished and balanced scalp. A healthy scalp not only promotes optimal hair growth but also ensures that the hair remains strong and vibrant. Essential oils can play a vital role in maintaining scalp health by addressing common issues like dandruff, dryness, and irritation.

Peppermint essential oil

Peppermint essential oil, derived from the peppermint plant, is known for its invigorating and cooling properties. It possesses antimicrobial and antifungal attributes, making it effective in combatting dandruff and other scalp conditions. Peppermint oil also improves circulation to the scalp, promoting hair growth and a refreshed scalp.

Tea tree essential oil

Tea tree essential oil, obtained from the leaves of the tea tree, is a powerhouse when it comes to scalp health. It possesses strong antiseptic properties that help combat scalp infections, dandruff, and even psoriasis. Tea tree oil also soothes itchiness and reduces redness, contributing to a healthier and more comfortable scalp.

Lavender essential oil

Lavender essential oil, as mentioned earlier, not only strengthens the hair but also contributes to a balanced scalp. Its gentle and calming properties help soothe scalp irritation and reduce inflammation. Lavender oil promotes a serene and nourished scalp, providing an ideal environment for hair growth and overall hair health.

To harness the benefits of these essential oils for scalp health, a soothing scalp massage oil can be created. Combining a few drops of peppermint, tea tree, and lavender essential oils with a carrier oil such as sweet almond or olive oil creates an effective blend. Massaging this blend into the scalp in a gentle, circular motion improves blood circulation, soothes the scalp, and promotes a healthy environment for hair growth.

CHAPTER 4

NATURAL PERFUMES AND FRAGRANCES

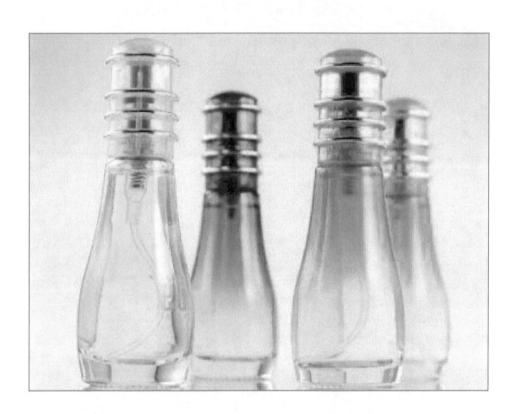

Fragrance, an invisible yet powerful element of our lives, holds the potential to transport us to another time, evoke memories, and influence our moods. Perfumes and fragrances are an integral part of our daily routines, and as our understanding of natural and holistic approaches to wellness deepens, the appeal of natural perfumes crafted with essential oils continues to grow. In this chapter, we embark on a journey into the world of natural perfumes and fragrances, exploring the art of blending essential oils to create unique and alluring scents that resonate with our individuality and offer a sustainable and harmonious alternative to conventional perfumery.

The Art of Blending Essential Oils for Perfumes

Creating a natural perfume using essential oils is an art form that requires a keen understanding of the aromatic properties, volatility, and intensity of each oil. Unlike synthetic fragrances, natural perfumes harness the true essence of botanicals, capturing the nuances and complexities of their scents. To begin crafting a natural perfume, one must grasp the fundamentals of blending essential oils to achieve a balanced and harmonious fragrance.

Each essential oil is characterized by its unique top, middle, and base notes. The top notes are the initial scents perceived upon application, typically citrusy and fresh. Middle notes emerge shortly after, offering a transition between the top and base notes, often floral or spicy. Base notes are the deep and lingering scents that anchor the fragrance and become more pronounced over time, often woody or resinous.

When blending essential oils for a perfume, a perfumer carefully selects oils from each note category, considering their olfactory profile, intensity, and how they interact with one another. The goal is to achieve a well-rounded perfume that unfolds gracefully, captivating the senses from the first application to the lasting impressions.

The Olfactory Palette: Aromatic Families of Essential Oils

Essential oils can be categorized into aromatic families based on their olfactory characteristics and chemical composition. These families serve as a guide for perfumers, assisting in creating synergistic and complementary blends. Let us explore some prominent aromatic families and their distinctive features.

Floral Aromatic Family

Floral essential oils are derived from various flowers and blossoms, offering a wide spectrum of scents from delicate and powdery to rich and opulent. Examples of floral essential oils include rose, jasmine, lavender, and ylang-ylang. These oils are often used as middle or top notes in perfumery, lending a romantic and elegant touch to the fragrance.

Citrus Aromatic Family

Citrus essential oils are extracted from the peels of citrus fruits, presenting vibrant and uplifting scents. Lemon, orange, grapefruit, and bergamot are classic examples of citrus oils. They predominantly serve as top notes, imparting a refreshing and invigorating aroma to the perfume.

Woody Aromatic Family

Woody essential oils emanate earthy, grounding, and often masculine scents. Cedarwood, sandalwood, pine, and vetiver are typical representatives of this family. Wood oils are primarily base or middle notes, adding depth and longevity to the fragrance.

Spicy Aromatic Family

Spicy essential oils exude warmth, depth, and a hint of exoticism. Commonly used as middle notes, oils like cinnamon, clove, cardamom, and black pepper impart a spicy and alluring character to the perfume, making it more captivating and intriguing.

Herbal Aromatic Family

Herbal essential oils are derived from various herbs and plants, presenting fresh, aromatic, and sometimes medicinal scents. Lavender, rosemary, basil, and peppermint are examples of herbal oils. They are versatile and can serve as top, middle, or base notes, depending on the composition of the fragrance.

Understanding the aromatic families allows perfumers to select oils that complement one another, facilitating the creation of well-balanced and captivating natural perfumes.

The Importance of Scent Layering

Layering is a crucial aspect of creating a natural perfume that unfolds beautifully and lasts throughout the day. It involves applying different scents to various pulse points on the body, allowing the fragrance to develop and interact uniquely with an individual's skin chemistry.

When layering a natural perfume, it's common to start with lighter, more volatile top notes applied on areas such as the wrists, neck, and behind the ears. As these top notes dissipate, the middle and base notes emerge, creating a multi-dimensional olfactory experience.

Moreover, considering the variability of skin chemistry among individuals, the same perfume can manifest differently in each person. Skin type, pH levels, and body temperature influence how the perfume interacts with the skin, resulting in a unique and personalized fragrance for each wearer.

Sustainable and Ethical Perfumery with Essential Oils

In recent times, sustainability and ethical practices have become paramount in various industries, including perfumery. Consumers are increasingly conscious of the environmental and ethical impact of their choices, leading to a surge in demand for sustainably sourced and cruelty-free fragrances.

Natural perfumery using essential oils aligns with these values, as it often involves responsibly sourcing botanicals and utilizing eco-friendly extraction methods. Essential oils are typically obtained through steam distillation or cold-press extraction, methods that are gentle on the environment and preserve the plant's natural essence.

Moreover, the move towards sustainable practices extends to the packaging of natural perfumes. Many perfumers opt for recyclable and biodegradable materials for their packaging, reducing waste and minimizing their ecological footprint.

Ethical considerations also encompass ensuring fair trade practices and supporting local communities involved in the cultivation and extraction of essential oils. By choosing natural perfumes crafted with ethical values in mind, consumers can embrace fragrances that not only enrich their senses but also contribute positively to the planet and its inhabitants.

Crafting Your Signature Scent: A Personalized Journey

The world of natural perfumery invites individuals to embark on a personal and artistic journey in discovering and creating their signature scents. Unlike mass-produced perfumes that offer uniform fragrances to the masses, natural perfumes allow for a level of customization that resonates with individual preferences and personalities.

Perfume enthusiasts can experiment with various essential oils, combining different notes and aromatic families to create a fragrance that aligns with their unique identity. This personalized approach ensures that the perfume harmonizes with one's natural body chemistry, resulting in a scent that feels intrinsically 'you.'

In this creative process, individuals can document their blends, refine their preferences, and curate a collection of signature scents for different moods, occasions, or seasons. Crafting a personalized perfume becomes an intimate and enjoyable endeavor, epitomizing the true essence of natural perfumery.

Natural perfumes and fragrances crafted with essential oils offer a compelling alternative to synthetic fragrances, aligning with the growing global shift towards sustainability, wellness, and ethical consumerism. The art of blending essential oils to create unique and captivating scents allows individuals to embrace their distinctiveness and enjoy the therapeutic benefits of aromatherapy simultaneously.

BOOK 5

AROMATHERAPY FOR RELAXATION AND SLEEP

CHAPTER 1

CREATING A RELAXING ATMOSPHERE

(AROMATHERAPY DIFFUSERS, CANDLES)

In the hustle and bustle of our modern lives, finding solace and relaxation can be a challenge. Our day-to-day routines, responsibilities, and the constant onslaught of technology can leave us feeling stressed and overwhelmed. It is in these moments that the ancient practice of aromatherapy comes to our aid, offering a natural and holistic way to induce relaxation and cultivate a calming atmosphere. In this chapter, we will delve into the art and science of creating a relaxing atmosphere through aromatherapy. We will explore the use of aromatherapy diffusers and aromatic candles, understanding their benefits and applications in setting up an environment that nurtures relaxation and tranquility.

Aromatherapy Diffusers

Aromatherapy diffusers are versatile devices that play a crucial role in setting the stage for a relaxing atmosphere. These devices allow for the dispersal of essential oils into the air, utilizing their aromatic properties to influence our mood and state of mind. The therapeutic molecules released by essential oils interact with our olfactory system, affecting our brain and emotional responses.

Types of Aromatherapy Diffusers

There are various types of aromatherapy diffusers, each employing distinct mechanisms to disperse essential oils effectively. Understanding the differences and advantages of each type is vital in choosing the right diffuser for specific needs and preferences.

Ultrasonic Diffusers

Ultrasonic diffusers are popular for their ability to disperse a fine mist of water and essential oils into the air. The device uses ultrasonic vibrations to break down the essential oil and water into tiny particles, resulting in a delicate mist that is released into the room. This mist not only carries the aroma of the essential oil but also has a humidifying effect, making it especially beneficial in dry environments. Ultrasonic diffusers are gentle, preserving the therapeutic properties of the oils as they do not use heat in the process.

Nebulizing Diffusers

Nebulizing diffusers are known for their efficiency in delivering pure essential oil into the air. These diffusers do not require water or heat; instead, they atomize the essential oil directly, creating a concentrated and potent mist of particles. Since nebulizing diffusers do not dilute the essential oils, they retain their full therapeutic benefits. This type of diffuser is excellent for those seeking a strong and immediate aromatic experience.

Evaporative Diffusers

Evaporative diffusers function by using a fan to blow air through a pad or filter soaked with essential oils. As the air passes over the pad, it evaporates the oils, dispersing their aroma into the room. While evaporative diffusers are simple and affordable, they may not provide as strong or consistent a fragrance as other types. However, they are still effective in spreading essential oil scents throughout a room.

Heat Diffusers

Heat diffusers utilize a heat source, often a candle or an electric element, to gently warm the essential oils, causing them to evaporate into the air. While this method effectively releases the aroma of the oils, it can alter their chemical composition and diminish their therapeutic properties. Heat diffusers are a good option for those seeking a subtle and continuous dispersion of essential oil scents.

Aromatic Candles

Aromatic candles have been cherished for generations as a means to create a soothing and inviting ambiance. The combination of soft, flickering light and gentle aromas emitted by these candles provides a multi-sensory experience that calms the mind and alleviates stress. Aromatherapy candles are crafted using natural essential oils, allowing for a purer and more therapeutic aroma.

Types of Aromatic Candles:

There is a wide array of aromatic candles available, each designed to cater to specific preferences and purposes. Understanding the types of aromatic candles aids in choosing the most suitable one to enhance relaxation and create a calming atmosphere.

Soy Wax Candles:

Soy wax candles are made from soybean oil, making them a popular choice for those seeking a more eco-friendly and sustainable option. They burn cleaner and longer than traditional paraffin wax candles and have a lower melting point, allowing the aroma of the essential oils to diffuse more effectively. Soy wax candles can be infused with various essential oils to create a relaxing ambiance.

Beeswax Candles

Beeswax candles are crafted from the wax produced by bees. They have a natural, honey-like aroma and emit negative ions when burned, which can help purify the air. Beeswax candles burn cleanly and slowly, providing a long-lasting and soothing aromatic experience.

Paraffin Wax Candles

Paraffin wax candles are the most common type of candles and are widely available. However, they are made from petroleum by-products and may release harmful chemicals when burned. It is advisable to opt for natural wax candles like soy or beeswax for a healthier and more aromatic choice.

Aroma Combinations and Benefits

Aromatic candles often come in various scents and combinations, each with its unique benefits. Lavender, chamomile, eucalyptus, and citrus scents are commonly used in aromatherapy candles for their relaxing and mood-enhancing properties. Understanding the effects of different aromas allows individuals to choose candles that align with their relaxation goals and preferences.

Safety and Proper Usage:

While aromatic candles can create a serene atmosphere, it is crucial to prioritize safety when using them. Always follow the manufacturer's instructions for lighting and extinguishing candles. Place candles on heat-resistant surfaces and away from flammable materials. Never leave a burning candle unattended, and ensure that they are fully extinguished before leaving a room.

Combining Aromatherapy Diffusers and Candles

To create a truly immersive and relaxing atmosphere, combining aromatherapy diffusers with aromatic candles can be highly effective. This combination provides both a visual and olfactory delight, enhancing the overall ambiance and promoting a deep sense of relaxation. Utilizing both diffusers and candles also allows for a consistent and prolonged diffusion of essential oils into the environment.

By strategically placing diffusers and candles throughout a space, individuals can tailor the aroma to suit their preferences, making the atmosphere more inviting and tranquil. The interplay between the calming flicker of candlelight and the soothing scents of essential oils adds a layer of comfort and serenity to any setting, whether it's a cozy bedroom, a peaceful living room, or a spa-like bathroom.

CHAPTER 2

CALMING BLENDS FOR ANXIETY AND STRESS

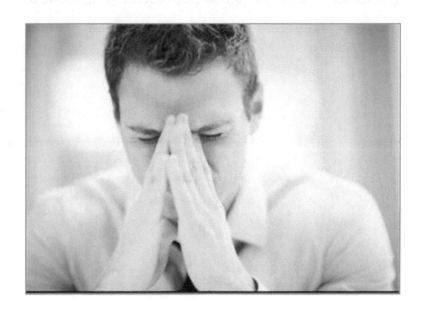

Stress and anxiety are omnipresent in today's fast-paced world, affecting millions of individuals worldwide. The constant demands of work, personal responsibilities, and the pressures of daily life can take a toll on mental and emotional well-being. Fortunately, aromatherapy offers a holistic and natural approach to managing these challenges, offering relief and promoting a sense of calm and relaxation. In this chapter, we will delve deeply into the world of calming blends for anxiety and stress, exploring the essential oils and blending techniques that can be employed to create powerful and effective remedies.

Essential Oils for Anxiety and Stress

Essential oils are the heart and soul of aromatherapy, each possessing unique aromatic compounds that influence emotions, mood, and overall well-being. When it comes to managing anxiety and stress, selecting the right essential oils is crucial. Here, we will explore some of the most potent and soothing essential oils that have proven effective in alleviating stress and anxiety.

Lavender Oil

Lavender (Lavandula angustifolia) is perhaps the most well-known and widely used essential oil for calming nerves and reducing anxiety. Its sweet, floral aroma is instantly recognizable and is known to promote relaxation, ease tension, and improve sleep quality. Lavender oil's versatility makes it a staple in any calming blend. It can be used alone or in combination with other essential oils to enhance its effectiveness.

Chamomile Oil

Chamomile (Matricaria chamomilla or Chamaemelum nobile) is another excellent choice for soothing anxiety and stress. Roman chamomile and German chamomile are the two most common varieties used in aromatherapy. Chamomile oil possesses a gentle, apple-like scent and is prized for its calming and sedative properties. It is often used to alleviate nervousness, restlessness, and irritability.

Bergamot Oil

Bergamot (Citrus bergamia) is a citrus oil with a bright, uplifting scent. Despite its invigorating aroma, bergamot oil is remarkably effective in reducing anxiety. It can promote relaxation while simultaneously elevating mood and reducing feelings of depression. Bergamot is a top note in aromatherapy, making it an excellent addition to blends.

Frankincense Oil

Frankincense (Boswellia carterii) has a deep, resinous aroma that is both grounding and spiritually uplifting. This oil is renowned for its ability to induce a sense of tranquility and peace, making it a valuable ally in managing stress. Frankincense also has the added benefit of promoting deep and focused breathing, which can be particularly helpful in stressful situations.

Ylang-Ylang Oil

Ylang-ylang (Cananga odorata) has a rich, exotic floral scent that is both sensual and soothing. This oil is known for its ability to reduce feelings of nervousness and tension. Ylang-ylang is often used to address emotional imbalances, promoting a sense of inner calm and relaxation.

Patchouli Oil

Patchouli (Pogostemon cablin) has a distinct earthy and musky aroma. While it may not be everyone's favorite scent, patchouli is a powerful oil for grounding and calming the mind. It is especially beneficial for individuals experiencing anxiety related to overthinking or mental restlessness.

Marjoram Oil

Marjoram (Origanum majorana) has a warm and herbaceous aroma that is incredibly comforting. This oil is known for its ability to ease muscle tension and promote relaxation. It is particularly effective in blends designed to alleviate physical symptoms of stress, such as muscle stiffness.

Clary Sage Oil

Clary sage (Salvia sclarea) has a sweet and herbaceous scent. This oil is renowned for its calming and euphoric properties. It can help balance hormones, making it useful for managing anxiety related to hormonal fluctuations, such as PMS or menopause.

Geranium Oil

Geranium (Pelargonium graveolens) has a floral and slightly fruity aroma. It is known for its balancing and calming effects on the mind and emotions. Geranium oil can help reduce feelings of tension and anxiety while promoting emotional stability.

Vetiver Oil

Vetiver (Vetiveria zizanioides) has a deep, earthy, and grounding aroma. This oil is excellent for individuals who find themselves "in their heads" too much, as it helps anchor the mind to the present moment. Vetiver oil is also helpful for improving sleep quality.

Blending Techniques

Creating the perfect calming blend is both an art and a science. It involves understanding the unique characteristics of each essential oil and how they interact with one another. To craft an effective blend, consider the following blending techniques:

Base, Middle, and Top Notes

Essential oils are categorized into base, middle, and top notes based on their volatility and aroma. Understanding these categories is fundamental to creating a well-balanced blend.

Base Notes

These oils are the heaviest and slowest to evaporate. They provide the foundation and longevity of the blend. Examples include patchouli, frankincense, and vetiver.

Middle Notes

Middle note oils have a balanced rate of evaporation and act as the body of the blend. They contribute to the overall scent and therapeutic properties. Examples include lavender, chamomile, and geranium.

Top Notes

Top note oils are the most volatile and provide the initial aroma of the blend. They are often uplifting and energizing. Examples include bergamot, ylang-ylang, and clary sage.

Synergy

Synergy refers to the harmonious interaction between different essential oils in a blend. When combined thoughtfully, essential oils can enhance each other's therapeutic properties. For example, blending lavender (a middle note) with bergamot (a top note) can create a calming blend that is both uplifting and relaxing.

Ratio

The proportion of each essential oil in a blend can significantly impact its overall effectiveness. A common ratio for a calming blend might be 2 drops of lavender (middle note), 1 drop of frankincense (base note), and 1 drop of bergamot (top note). However, ratios can vary based on personal preference and intended use.

Dilution

Essential oils are potent and should be diluted before applying them to the skin. Carrier oils, such as jojoba, sweet almond, or coconut oil, are often used to dilute essential oils. The recommended dilution ratio is typically 1-3% for adults, but it may vary depending on individual sensitivity and the purpose of the blend.

Patch Testing

Before applying a blend to a larger area of the body, it's essential to conduct a patch test to check for any allergic reactions or skin sensitivities. Apply a small amount of the diluted blend to a small patch of skin (e.g., the inner forearm) and monitor for any adverse reactions.

Creating the perfect blend often involves some trial and error. It's advisable to start with small batches and experiment with different combinations and ratios of essential oils until you find a blend that resonates with you.

CHAPTER 3

PROMOTING BETTER SLEEP

(SEDATIVE OILS, BEDTIME RITUALS)

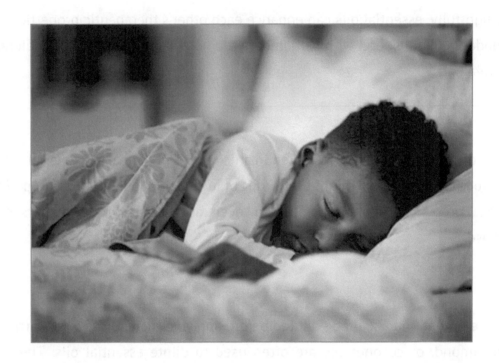

Quality sleep is the cornerstone of overall health and well-being. However, in our fast-paced and often stressful lives, many individuals struggle with insomnia, restless nights, or difficulty falling asleep. Aromatherapy offers a natural and non-invasive approach to promote better sleep and improve the overall quality of rest. In this chapter, we will delve into the various aspects of using aromatherapy to enhance sleep, including the use of sedative essential oils and the incorporation of bedtime rituals.

Sedative Essential Oils

Sedative essential oils play a vital role in creating an environment conducive to sleep. These oils possess unique properties that can induce relaxation, calm the mind, and prepare the body for restorative rest. By understanding the qualities of sedative essential oils and how they influence sleep patterns, individuals can harness the power of aromatherapy to enhance their sleep quality.

Lavender: The Universal Sleep Aid

Lavender essential oil is perhaps the most well-known and widely used essential oil for promoting better sleep. With its gentle and soothing aroma, lavender has a remarkable ability to reduce anxiety, lower stress levels, and induce a state of calmness. Numerous scientific studies have confirmed lavender's efficacy in improving sleep quality and reducing the time it takes to fall asleep.

The key to using lavender essential oil for sleep is to diffuse it in the bedroom before bedtime. A few drops in an aromatherapy diffuser will release its calming scent into the air, creating a tranquil atmosphere that invites relaxation. Alternatively, a drop or two on a pillow or a cloth near the pillow can have a similar effect.

Chamomile: Nature's Tranquilizer

Chamomile essential oil is another excellent choice for those seeking restful sleep. Chamomile is renowned for its calming and sedative properties, making it an ideal remedy for sleeplessness caused by anxiety or racing thoughts. This gentle oil is known to alleviate tension and soothe the nervous system.

To use chamomile essential oil for sleep, a few drops can be added to a warm bath before bedtime, allowing the soothing aroma to envelop you as you soak. Alternatively, it can be combined with carrier oil and massaged onto the skin or used in a room spray to create a relaxing environment.

Marjoram: Muscle Relaxation for Deeper Sleep

Marjoram essential oil is particularly beneficial for individuals who experience muscle tension or physical discomfort that hinders their sleep. This oil possesses muscle relaxant properties, which can help alleviate physical tension and promote a more comfortable and restful sleep.

To utilize marjoram essential oil for sleep, it can be added to a carrier oil and gently massaged onto areas of the body where tension is present, such as the neck, shoulders, and lower back. The calming effect of marjoram can ease physical discomfort and contribute to a deeper and more peaceful slumber.

Sandalwood: A Grounding and Calming Essence

Sandalwood essential oil is revered for its grounding and calming properties, making it an excellent choice for individuals who struggle with racing thoughts or a restless mind before bedtime. Sandalwood's earthy and woody aroma can help anchor the mind and induce a sense of inner peace.

To incorporate sandalwood essential oil into your sleep routine, it can be diffused in the bedroom or diluted in carrier oil and applied to the pulse points, such as the wrists and temples. This will enable you to benefit from its tranquilizing effects, facilitating a more serene and undisturbed night's sleep.

Bergamot: Uplifting and Relaxing

Bergamot essential oil is unique in its ability to simultaneously uplift and relax the mind. It is particularly beneficial for individuals who may be feeling emotionally drained or anxious and need a gentle mood boost along with relaxation to fall asleep peacefully.

To use bergamot essential oil for sleep, it can be diffused in the bedroom to create a balanced atmosphere. Its citrusy and floral notes can help alleviate stress and elevate the mood, creating a more harmonious mental state conducive to restful sleep.

Bedtime Rituals

Incorporating aromatherapy into your bedtime rituals can serve as a powerful signal to your body that it's time to unwind and prepare for sleep. Establishing a consistent routine that involves the use of essential oils can enhance the effectiveness of aromatherapy in promoting relaxation and better sleep.

Aromatic Bath Rituals

Taking a warm, aromatic bath before bedtime is a luxurious and effective way to prepare both the body and mind for sleep. Aromatherapy bath rituals can help relax tense muscles, soothe the nervous system, and create a sense of tranquility.

To create an aromatic bath ritual, simply add a few drops of your chosen sedative essential oil (such as lavender or chamomile) to a carrier oil, milk, or Epsom salts, and then add this mixture to your bathwater. As you soak in the fragrant water, allow your worries to melt away and focus on the sensory experience. The warmth, the scent, and the relaxation all contribute to a serene state that encourages a peaceful night's sleep.

Bedtime Diffusion

Using an aromatherapy diffuser in the bedroom before sleep is a delightful way to create a calming atmosphere. Diffusing sedative essential oils like lavender or marjoram can transform your bedroom into a sanctuary of relaxation.

Set up your diffuser on a stable surface, ensuring it's safe and easy to use. Add the recommended number of drops of your chosen essential oil(s), and let the diffuser work its magic. As you climb into bed, the room will be filled with a soothing aroma, gently coaxing you into a peaceful slumber.

Massage with Essential Oils

Aromatherapy massage can be a beautiful addition to your bedtime routine, promoting relaxation and helping you unwind after a long day. Using diluted sedative essential oils, such as lavender or sandalwood, for massage can further enhance the calming effect.

Create a massage oil blend by diluting the chosen essential oil(s) in a carrier oil like sweet almond oil or jojoba oil. Apply this blend to your body, focusing on areas where tension tends to accumulate, such as the neck, shoulders, and feet. The combination of touch and aroma can induce deep relaxation, making it easier to transition into a peaceful sleep.

Creating a Sleep-Inducing Atmosphere

Transforming your bedroom into a sleep-inducing sanctuary can greatly influence the quality of your sleep. This involves decluttering your sleeping space, choosing calming colors and textures, and incorporating aromatherapy elements.

Consider using soft, breathable bedding, blackout curtains, and comfortable pillows to create a cozy sleep environment. In addition to using essential oil diffusers, you can place sachets of dried lavender or chamomile near your pillow or under your mattress for a subtle, soothing aroma. The combination of a comfortable setting and aromatherapy can make your bedroom the ideal place for restorative sleep.

CHAPTER 4

STRESS REDUCTION TECHNIQUES

(BREATHING EXERCISES, MEDITATION)

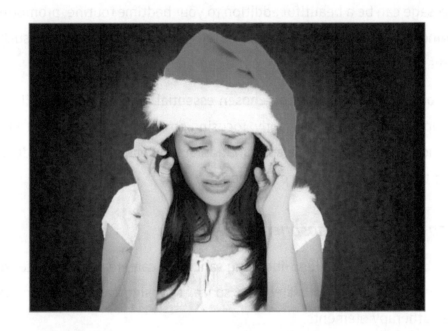

I n the hustle and bustle of modern life, stress has become an unwelcome companion for many. It's essential to equip ourselves with effective stress reduction techniques to maintain mental and physical well-being. This chapter explores various stress reduction techniques, emphasizing the integration of aromatherapy to amplify their benefits and promote a calmer, more balanced state of mind.

Breathing Exercises

Breathing is an involuntary action that sustains life, yet it's often taken for granted. Deliberate, mindful breathing exercises have the power to transform how we feel and manage stress. The beauty of breathing exercises lies in their simplicity and accessibility; anyone can practice them anytime, anywhere.

Diaphragmatic Breathing

Diaphragmatic breathing, also known as deep belly breathing or abdominal breathing, is a foundational breathing technique used to promote relaxation and reduce stress. In this technique, you focus on engaging your diaphragm rather than shallow breathing into your chest.

Begin by finding a comfortable, quiet place to sit or lie down. Place one hand on your chest and the other on your abdomen. Inhale slowly through your nose, allowing your abdomen to expand like a balloon. Feel the breath move into your lower lungs and push your hand on your abdomen out. Exhale slowly through your mouth, allowing your abdomen to contract.

Practice diaphragmatic breathing for a few minutes each day, gradually increasing the duration as you become more comfortable with the technique. This practice can calm the nervous system, reduce muscle tension, and promote a sense of calm and centeredness, making it an ideal stress reduction tool.

Box Breathing

Box breathing, also known as square breathing, is a technique that involves a rhythmic and structured pattern of breath. It's named "box" because each phase of the breath (inhale, hold, exhale, hold) is typically counted to a consistent number, creating a square-like pattern.

Start by finding a quiet space and sitting or lying down comfortably. Close your eyes and take a slow, deep breath in for a count of four. Hold your breath for a count of four. Exhale slowly for a count of four. Hold your breath again for a count of four. Repeat this cycle for a few minutes, maintaining a steady and even rhythm.

Box breathing helps regulate the autonomic nervous system, bringing a sense of balance and reducing stress and anxiety. Integrating aromatic essential oils during this exercise, perhaps through a diffuser or inhalation, can enhance the relaxing effect, making the practice even more beneficial.

Progressive Muscle Relaxation (PMR) with Aromatherapy

Progressive Muscle Relaxation (PMR) is a technique that involves tensing and relaxing specific muscle groups to release physical tension. By combining PMR with aromatherapy, we can further augment its stress-relieving effects.

Find a quiet and comfortable space to sit or lie down. Begin by tensing a muscle group (e.g., hands, shoulders, or legs) for a few seconds, then release the tension while taking a deep breath in. As you exhale, let go of any remaining tension in that muscle group. Repeat this process for each muscle group, progressing from head to toe.

Using calming essential oils like lavender, chamomile, or bergamot in a diffuser or through a gentle massage can deepen the relaxation response during PMR. The soothing aroma complements the physical relaxation, creating a powerful synergy that reduces stress and promotes a profound sense of calm.

Meditation

Meditation is a centuries-old practice that involves focusing the mind on a particular object, thought, or activity to achieve a state of mental clarity, tranquility, and mindfulness. It is a powerful tool for stress reduction and emotional well-being, and when combined with aromatherapy, its benefits are elevated.

Mindfulness Meditation

Mindfulness meditation is a form of meditation that emphasizes being fully present in the moment observing thoughts and sensations without judgment. It cultivates awareness of the present moment and can help alleviate stress by calming the mind.

To practice mindfulness meditation, find a quiet and comfortable space. Sit or lie down in a relaxed position. Close your eyes and bring your attention to your breath. Notice the sensation of the breath as it enters and leaves your nostrils or the rise and fall of your chest or abdomen. If your mind wanders, gently bring your focus back to your breath.

Integrating the gentle aromas of essential oils into your meditation space can enhance the sensory experience, aiding in relaxation and deepening your meditative state. Choose oils like frankincense, lavender, or sandalwood, known for their calming and grounding properties, and use a diffuser to disperse the scent throughout the room.

Guided Imagery Meditation

Guided imagery meditation involves mentally visualizing a peaceful and serene scene or scenario to induce relaxation and reduce stress. It's a technique that engages the power of imagination to promote a state of tranquility.

To practice guided imagery meditation, start by finding a comfortable and quiet space. Close your eyes and take a few deep, calming breaths. Imagine a place or scenario that brings you peace and joy, such as a tranquil beach, a forest, or a meadow. Engage all your senses in this visualization—what you see, hear, smell, and feel. Allow yourself to immerse in this mental oasis, leaving behind any stress or worry.

Introducing the aromatic essence of essential oils during guided imagery can deepen the sensory experience, transporting you to the imagined peaceful place more vividly. Select oils like lavender, cedarwood, or bergamot to complement your chosen scene and use a diffuser to diffuse the aroma, enhancing the meditation's effectiveness.

BOOK 6

CREATING A
HOLISTIC HOME ENVIRONMENT

CHAPTER 1

NATURAL CLEANING
WITH ESSENTIAL OILS

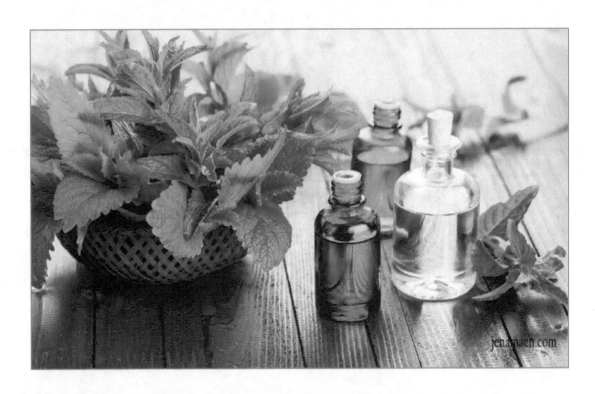

In our quest to create a holistic home environment that promotes overall well-being, one of the fundamental aspects to consider is adopting natural cleaning practices. Conventional cleaning products are often laden with harsh chemicals that can have detrimental effects on both our health and the environment. In contrast, essential oils, derived from plants and possessing powerful natural cleaning properties, offer a safe, effective, and eco-friendly alternative that not only cleans but also leaves behind a refreshing and pleasant scent. In this chapter, we will delve deep into the world of natural cleaning with essential oils, exploring their properties, applications, and the numerous benefits they bring to our homes.

Applications in Cleaning

Now that we have a foundational understanding of essential oils, let's explore how we can put them to practical use in our cleaning routines. Essential oils can be incorporated into various cleaning applications, allowing us to replace commercial cleaning products with natural and effective alternatives. Here are some key ways in which essential oils can be used in cleaning:

All-Purpose Cleaners: One of the simplest ways to use essential oils for cleaning is by creating your own all-purpose cleaner. Here's a basic recipe:

Ingredients:

- 2 cups distilled water
- 1/2 cup white vinegar
- 10-20 drops of essential oil (e.g., lavender, lemon, or tea tree)

Instructions:

1. Combine all the ingredients in a spray bottle.
2. Shake well before each use.
3. Spray on surfaces and wipe with a clean cloth or sponge.

This DIY all-purpose cleaner not only effectively cleans and disinfects but also leaves a delightful fragrance in its wake.

Disinfectants

Essential oils like tea tree, eucalyptus, and thyme have powerful antimicrobial properties. Adding a few drops of these oils to your cleaning solutions can help disinfect surfaces naturally. For instance, you can create a natural disinfectant by combining water, vinegar, and a few drops of tea tree oil.

Stain Removers

Essential oils can also be used to tackle stubborn stains. For example, lemon essential oil is excellent for removing grease stains, while a mixture of baking soda and tea tree oil can be effective for removing mold and mildew stains.

Deodorizers

Many commercial air fresheners merely mask odors and may contain harmful chemicals. Essential oils, on the other hand, can neutralize odors naturally. A few drops of your favorite essential oil, such as lavender or citrus, added to a small bowl of baking soda can be placed in closets or bathrooms to absorb and eliminate unpleasant odors.

Benefits of Natural Cleaning with Essential Oils

As we've seen, natural cleaning with essential oils offers a multitude of advantages. Let's delve deeper into these benefits to understand why this approach is gaining popularity among homeowners seeking a holistic home environment:

Safety

One of the most compelling reasons to choose natural cleaning with essential oils is safety. Commercial cleaning products often contain harsh chemicals like chlorine, ammonia, and formaldehyde, which can be harmful if ingested or if their fumes are inhaled. On the contrary, essential oils are derived from plants and are non-toxic when used as directed. This makes them safer for both your family and the environment.

Reduced Environmental Impact

Conventional cleaning products can have a significant environmental impact due to the production, use, and disposal of their chemical ingredients. Essential oils, being derived from renewable plant sources, have a far lower environmental footprint. Additionally, when used in homemade cleaning solutions, they reduce the need for single-use plastic bottles, further contributing to environmental sustainability.

Improved Indoor Air Quality

Many commercial cleaning products release volatile organic compounds (VOCs) into the air, which can contribute to indoor air pollution and have adverse health effects. In contrast, essential oils not only clean but also release pleasant fragrances into the air, improving indoor air quality and creating a more inviting atmosphere.

Versatility

The versatility of essential oils is another key benefit. With a wide array of essential oils available, you can customize your cleaning products to suit your preferences and cleaning needs. Whether you want a citrus-scented kitchen cleaner or a calming lavender-scented bathroom cleaner, essential oils offer endless possibilities.

Therapeutic Benefits

Apart from their cleaning prowess, essential oils also bring therapeutic benefits to your home environment. The aromas of essential oils can have a profound impact on mood and well-being. For instance, the scent of lavender promotes relaxation, while citrus oils like lemon and orange can uplift and energize your spirit. By incorporating essential oils into your cleaning routine, you're not just tidying up your home; you're also enhancing your mental and emotional state.

Cost-Effective

Creating your own natural cleaning products with essential oils can be cost-effective in the long run. While the initial investment in essential oils may seem higher than buying commercial cleaners, a few drops of essential oil go a long way. A single bottle of essential oil can last for months, making it a budget-friendly choice.

Essential Oil Safety Considerations

Before we conclude this chapter, it's essential to address some safety considerations when using essential oils for cleaning. While essential oils are generally safe, they are potent and should be handled with care:

Dilution

Essential oils should be diluted before applying them to surfaces or using them in cleaning solutions. Undiluted essential oils can be too strong and may cause skin irritation or damage surfaces.

Skin Contact

When handling essential oils, be cautious to avoid direct skin contact, especially if you have sensitive skin. If skin irritation occurs, wash the affected area with mild soap and water and discontinue use.

Inhalation

Inhaling essential oil vapors is generally safe and can even have therapeutic benefits. However, avoid inhaling essential oil directly from the bottle or applying it to your face. Instead, use diffusers or allow the scent to disperse naturally in your living space.

Storage

Store essential oils in a cool, dark place, away from direct sunlight and out of reach of children and pets. Proper storage helps preserve their potency and extends their shelf life.

Mixing

When creating DIY cleaning solutions, always follow recommended recipes and guidelines for mixing essential oils with other ingredients. Combining essential oils with incompatible substances can lead to adverse reactions.

In the quest to create a holistic home environment that prioritizes health, well-being, and sustainability, natural cleaning with essential oils emerges as a powerful and practical solution. Understanding the properties and diverse applications of essential oils empowers us to transition from harmful, chemical-laden cleaning products to safe, effective, and environmentally friendly alternatives. By embracing this natural approach, not only do we contribute to a safer living space, but we also elevate our overall quality of life, making our homes truly harmonious sanctuaries of well-being.

CHAPTER 2

AIR PURIFICATION AND FRESHENING

(ROOM SPRAYS, DIY AIR FILTERS)

Indoor air quality is a critical aspect of creating a holistic home environment. The air we breathe within our homes can have a significant impact on our health and overall well-being. Modern living often entails spending a significant portion of our time indoors, making it vital to focus on purifying and freshening the air we encounter daily. This chapter delves into the various techniques and methods to effectively purify and freshen the air within our living spaces, promoting a healthier and more pleasant atmosphere.

Understanding Indoor Air Pollution

Indoor air pollution refers to the presence or introduction of harmful pollutants in the air within buildings or homes. These pollutants can be particulate matter, chemicals, biological agents, or other harmful substances that can pose health risks to the occupants. Sources of indoor air pollution are diverse and can range from household items to external factors. Common sources include cigarette smoke, cooking emissions, cleaning products, furniture, carpets, paints, and building materials.

Inadequate ventilation and airtight construction in modern buildings can contribute to a build-up of indoor air pollutants. Over time, exposure to these pollutants can lead to respiratory issues, allergies, asthma, and other health problems. Understanding the sources and types of indoor air pollution is crucial to developing effective strategies for air purification and freshening.

Air Purification Techniques

To combat indoor air pollution and enhance the quality of the air we breathe within our homes, various air purification techniques can be employed. These techniques aim to remove or reduce pollutants from the air, ensuring a healthier living environment.

Air Purifiers

Air purifiers are devices designed to remove airborne particles and pollutants from the indoor air. They typically consist of a fan that draws in air and passes it through filters, capturing particles such as dust, pollen, pet dander, smoke, and other pollutants. The cleaned air is then released back into the room.

Air purifiers utilize different types of filters, including High-Efficiency Particulate Air (HEPA) filters, activated carbon filters, ozone generators, and ultraviolet (UV) light filters. HEPA filters are highly efficient in capturing small particles, while activated carbon filters adsorb odors and chemicals. UV light filters help kill bacteria and viruses. Choosing the right air purifier based on the specific indoor air quality concerns is essential for effective air purification.

Indoor Plants

Indoor plants have the natural ability to purify the air by absorbing pollutants and releasing oxygen. Certain plants can help filter common indoor air pollutants such as benzene, formaldehyde, trichloroethylene, and ammonia. Examples of air-purifying plants include the snake plant (Sansevieria), spider plant (Chlorophytum comosum), pothos (Epipremnum aureum), and peace lily (Spathiphyllum).

Strategically placing indoor plants in different rooms of the house can contribute to improving air quality. However, it's important to note that not all plants are suitable for indoor environments, and some can be toxic to pets. Careful consideration and research should be undertaken before selecting plants for air purification purposes.

DIY Air Filters

Creating do-it-yourself (DIY) air filters is a cost-effective and eco-friendly way to enhance air quality within the home. DIY air filters can be made using common household items like fans, air filters, and a simple frame. The fan pulls air through the filter, capturing particles and pollutants. Regularly replacing the filter ensures optimal performance.

DIY air filters can be customized based on specific air quality concerns, and they provide an affordable alternative to commercial air purifiers. Regular maintenance and filter replacements are key to ensuring the effectiveness of DIY air filters.

DIY Air Fresheners and Room Sprays

Apart from purifying the air, maintaining a fresh and pleasant ambiance within the home is equally important. Commercial air fresheners often contain harmful chemicals that can negatively impact indoor air quality. Creating DIY air fresheners and room sprays using natural ingredients and essential oils is a healthier and safer alternative.

Essential Oil Diffusers

Essential oil diffusers are popular devices used to disperse the aromatic molecules of essential oils into the air. They come in various types, including ultrasonic diffusers, nebulizing diffusers, evaporative diffusers, and heat diffusers. These diffusers break down the essential oils into fine mist particles, allowing them to stay suspended in the air for extended periods.

Essential oil diffusers not only spread a pleasant aroma but also provide the therapeutic benefits associated with the chosen essential oils. For example, lavender essential oil can promote relaxation and better sleep, while peppermint essential oil can enhance focus and mental clarity.

DIY Room Sprays

Creating DIY room sprays using essential oils is a simple and effective way to refresh the air and eliminate odors in different areas of the home. These room sprays can be tailored to suit individual preferences by combining various essential oils to achieve a desired scent profile.

To create a DIY room spray, a mixture of distilled water and a few drops of preferred essential oils is combined in a spray bottle. The spray can be used to freshen up the air in living spaces, bedrooms, and bathrooms or even on linens and upholstery. The natural and pleasant aroma of essential oils contributes to a more inviting and enjoyable home environment.

Ensuring a clean, fresh, and healthy living environment is paramount for our overall well-being. Air purification and freshening play a crucial role in achieving this objective. Understanding indoor air pollution and implementing effective air purification techniques, such as utilizing air purifiers, indoor plants, and DIY air filters, can significantly enhance the quality of the air we breathe. Additionally, incorporating DIY air fresheners and room sprays using essential oils provides a natural and pleasing fragrance, contributing to a more pleasant and inviting ambiance within our homes. By adopting these practices, we can create a holistic home environment that promotes optimal health, relaxation, and overall happiness for all its inhabitants.

CHAPTER 3

AROMATHERAPY DIFFUSION METHODS

(DIFFUSERS, REED DIFFUSERS)

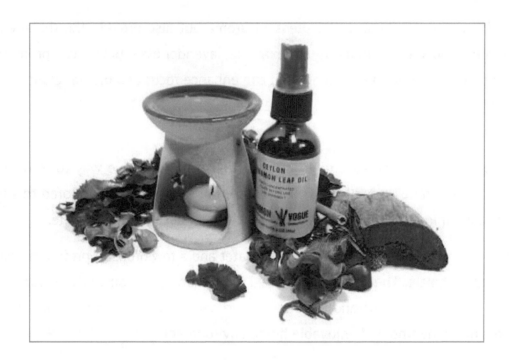

Aromatherapy, an age-old practice rooted in ancient civilizations, utilizes aromatic plant compounds to enhance physical, mental, and emotional well-being. The art of aromatherapy revolves around the utilization of essential oils, which are highly concentrated extracts obtained from various plants. These oils possess distinct fragrances and therapeutic properties that can be harnessed to create a tranquil and rejuvenating ambiance within our living spaces. One of the primary ways to incorporate the benefits of essential oils into our daily lives is through aromatherapy diffusion. This chapter explores the different methods of aromatherapy diffusion, providing insights into how each technique can be employed to elevate the atmosphere of our homes and promote a sense of calm and balance.

Understanding Aromatherapy Diffusion

Aromatherapy, with its origins dating back thousands of years, stands as a testament to the enduring allure and efficacy of natural remedies. At its core, aromatherapy involves the use of aromatic plant extracts, known as essential oils, to enhance well-being and promote health. The practice has evolved over the centuries and now encompasses various diffusion methods to disperse these essential oils into the air we breathe. Aromatherapy diffusion, the heart of this ancient practice, employs a range of techniques to disperse the aromatic molecules of essential oils, allowing us to experience their therapeutic benefits in a seamless and enjoyable manner.

The process of aromatherapy diffusion involves breaking down the essential oil into smaller particles and dispersing them into the air. These particles can be inhaled or absorbed through the skin, granting us access to the oil's inherent properties. Once inhaled, these aromatic molecules interact with our olfactory system, connecting with the brain's limbic system—the emotional center—triggering various responses that can influence our mood, emotions, and overall well-being.

Types of Aromatherapy Diffusion Methods

A diverse array of diffusion methods exists, each offering a unique approach to dispersing essential oils. Each method has its advantages, making them suitable for different settings and preferences. Let's delve into the various types of aromatherapy diffusion methods, exploring how they work and when to best utilize them.

Electric Diffusers

Electric diffusers stand out as one of the most popular and versatile types of diffusers available today. They utilize electricity to disperse essential oil molecules into the air. Typically, these diffusers combine essential oils with water to create a fine mist, which is then released into the environment.

One of the key benefits of electric diffusers is their ease of use. Users can control the intensity and duration of the diffusion, allowing for a tailored aromatherapy experience. Additionally, many electric diffusers feature LED lights, contributing to the ambiance of the room and creating a relaxing atmosphere.

Electric diffusers can be further categorized into ultrasonic, heat-based, and evaporative diffusers, each with its unique mechanism of action.

Ultrasonic Diffusers

Ultrasonic diffusers operate by using ultrasonic vibrations to break down essential oils into micro-particles. These particles are released into the air in the form of a fine mist, ensuring a gentle and consistent diffusion.

One of the notable advantages of ultrasonic diffusers is their ability to maintain the integrity of the essential oils' therapeutic properties. The oils are not heated during the process, preserving their natural qualities and ensuring maximum benefit.

Heat-Based Diffusers

Heat-based diffusers, as the name suggests, utilize heat to evaporate the essential oils into the air. This diffusion method often employs an external heat source, such as a candle or an electric heating element, to facilitate the process.

While heat-based diffusers are simple to use and provide an immediate release of aroma, it's essential to exercise caution, as heat can alter the chemical composition of the essential oils, potentially diminishing their therapeutic effects.

Evaporative Diffusers

Evaporative diffusers function by allowing essential oils to naturally evaporate into the air. Typically, a few drops of essential oil are applied to a pad or a similar absorbent material, and the oil gradually evaporates, diffusing the aroma into the surroundings.

This type of diffusion is commonly found in portable diffusers, such as those used in cars or as personal inhalers. It offers a convenient and portable way to experience aromatherapy on the go.

Nebulizing Diffusers

Nebulizing diffusers are revered for their potency and efficiency in dispersing essential oils. These diffusers use a pressurized air stream to atomize undiluted essential oil into tiny particles, which are then released into the air.

Unlike other diffusers, nebulizing diffusers do not require water or heat, ensuring that the essential oils retain their purest form and therapeutic properties. However, due to the direct dispersion of undiluted oil, they may consume oils more quickly.

Nebulizing diffusers are particularly beneficial for larger spaces, as they disperse a high concentration of essential oil particles, effectively covering a broader area.

Reed Diffusers

Reed diffusers offer a simple and elegant method of aromatherapy diffusion. They consist of a glass container filled with a blend of essential oils and a carrier liquid. Reeds made of materials like bamboo or rattan are placed in the container, absorbing the oil and diffusing its aroma into the surroundings.

One of the notable advantages of reed diffusers is their decorative aspect, adding a touch of sophistication to any space. Additionally, reed diffusers provide a constant, subtle diffusion of the chosen fragrance without the need for electricity or heat.

Steam Inhalation

Steam inhalation is a traditional method of aromatherapy diffusion. It involves adding a few drops of essential oil to a bowl of hot water and inhaling the steam. The steam carries the aromatic molecules of the oil, allowing them to reach the respiratory system.

This method is particularly effective for respiratory concerns and sinus congestion, providing quick relief. However, it's essential to exercise caution and maintain a safe distance to prevent burns from the hot steam.

Aromatherapy Jewelry

Aromatherapy jewelry, including necklaces, bracelets, and rings, serves as a wearable form of diffusion. These accessories are designed with small compartments or porous materials that hold essential oils. When worn, the body heat gently releases the aroma of the oils, allowing the wearer to experience aromatherapy benefits throughout the day.

Aromatherapy jewelry provides a convenient and personal way to enjoy the therapeutic effects of essential oils wherever you go.

Car Diffusers

Car diffusers are designed to fit into the car's ventilation system or use a USB port for power. They diffuse essential oils within the vehicle, creating a pleasant and refreshing environment during drives.

Car diffusers are particularly useful for promoting focus and reducing stress while driving, enhancing the overall driving experience.

Pottery or Terra Cotta Diffusers

Pottery or terra cotta diffusers are porous clay-based materials designed to absorb and diffuse essential oils. A few drops of essential oil are applied to the surface of the pottery, and the oil gradually evaporates, releasing the aroma into the air.

This method offers a natural and subtle diffusion, making it suitable for smaller spaces or areas where a gentle and continuous fragrance is desired.

Candle Diffusers

Candle diffusers combine the soothing ambiance of candlelight with the benefits of aromatherapy diffusion. The diffuser typically consists of a bowl or tray where water and a few drops of essential oil are placed. A candle is lit beneath the bowl, heating the water and causing the essential oil to evaporate and diffuse into the air.

While candle diffusers create a cozy atmosphere, it's important to use caution and never leave a lit candle unattended.

Spray or Room Sprays

Room sprays, also known as spritzers or mists, are a quick and convenient way to disperse essential oils into the air. They typically consist of a blend of water and essential oils, which can be sprayed into the air to refresh and aromatize a room.

Room sprays are perfect for immediate aromatherapy, allowing you to customize the fragrance in any space.

Choosing the Right Diffuser

Selecting the appropriate diffuser depends on several factors, including the size of the space, the desired intensity of diffusion, the specific benefits sought, and personal preferences. Here are some guidelines to help you choose the right diffuser for your needs:

Room Size

For larger rooms, nebulizing diffusers or electric diffusers are more effective due to their ability to disperse a higher concentration of essential oil particles over a broader area.

Intensity of Diffusion

If you prefer a subtle and consistent diffusion, ultrasonic diffusers or reed diffusers are ideal. For a more intense and immediate diffusion, nebulizing diffusers or steam inhalation may be more suitable.

Safety Considerations

If safety is a concern, especially if you have young children or pets, reed diffusers, ultrasonic diffusers, or electric diffusers are safer options compared to heat-based diffusers or candle diffusers.

Purpose of Diffusion

Consider the purpose of aromatherapy—whether it's for relaxation, concentration, respiratory support, or simply adding a pleasant aroma to the environment. Different diffusers may serve different purposes more effectively.

Tips for Effective Aromatherapy Diffusion

1. Always use high-quality, pure essential oils for aromatherapy diffusion. Choose oils from reputable sources to ensure their authenticity and therapeutic benefits.
2. When using diffusers that require dilution with water, follow the manufacturer's instructions and recommended dilution ratios to maintain the optimal balance and effectiveness of the essential oils.
3. Clean your diffuser regularly to prevent any buildup or residue. A clean diffuser ensures the diffusion process is efficient and maintains the quality of the essential oils.
4. Don't hesitate to experiment with different essential oil blends to discover the scents and combinations that resonate with you. Blending oils can create unique aromas and therapeutic effects.
5. Be mindful of the duration and frequency of diffusion. Avoid continuous and excessive diffusion, as it's important to give your body breaks and prevent olfactory fatigue.

Aromatherapy diffusion methods offer a gateway to experience the myriad benefits of essential oils in a convenient and enjoyable manner. The art and science of aromatherapy have been refined over centuries, culminating in a diverse range of diffusion techniques that cater to different preferences and settings. Whether you opt for the gentle mist of an ultrasonic diffuser, the elegance of reed diffusers, or the potency of nebulizing diffusers, each method has its own charm and effectiveness. By incorporating aromatherapy diffusion into our daily lives, we open the doors to a world of soothing fragrances and holistic well-being, transforming our living spaces into sanctuaries of health and tranquility. Experiment with various diffusion methods, embrace the natural scents of essential oils and let the aromatic molecules guide you toward a harmonious and balanced life.

CHAPTER 4

ENHANCING AMBIANCE WITH SCENT
(AROMATHERAPY CANDLES, POTPOURRI)

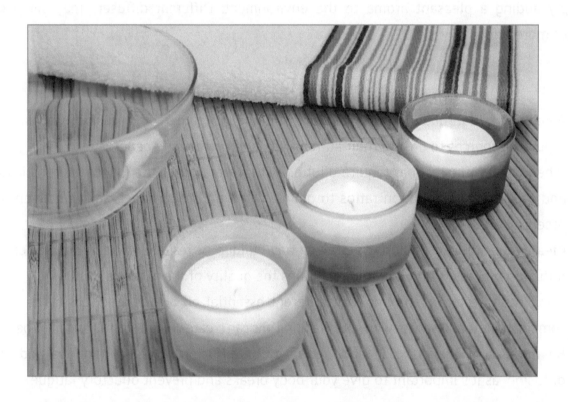

The scent is a powerful force in our lives. It has the ability to trigger memories, evoke emotions, and create a certain ambiance within a space. In the realm of holistic home environments, leveraging the power of scent is a fundamental aspect. By carefully choosing and strategically utilizing scents in our living spaces, we can enhance the ambiance, influence our mood, and ultimately craft an environment that resonates with our well-being. In this chapter, we will explore different methods to enhance ambiance through scent, including aromatherapy candles and potpourri.

Aromatherapy Candles: Illuminating Fragrance

Aromatherapy candles, often referred to as "illuminating fragrances," are a beacon in the world of holistic home environments. They play a significant role in not only emitting pleasing scents but also in providing therapeutic benefits through carefully chosen essential oils. As we delve deeper into the art of aromatherapy candles, we unveil the secrets of crafting them, choosing the right essential oils, understanding the benefits they offer, and the nuanced ways they influence our moods and atmosphere.

Crafting Aromatherapy Candles: The Artistry in Wax

Crafting aromatherapy candles is a delightful blend of art and science. It's a process where creativity meets precision to ensure the final product carries the desired scent and therapeutic properties. To start, one must gather the essential components: wax, wicks, fragrance (essential oils), a melting pot, a thermometer, and a suitable container or mold.

Wax Choices: The Foundation of Your Candle

The choice of wax is pivotal in candle making. Soy wax, derived from soybean oil, is a popular choice due to its eco-friendliness, clean burn, and ability to hold a good amount of fragrance. Beeswax, a natural byproduct of bees, is known for its subtle, honey-like aroma and natural purifying properties. Paraffin wax, though less preferred due to its petroleum base, is still widely used for its ability to hold fragrance well and give a smooth finish to candles.

Essential Oils: The Fragrant Heartbeat

Essential oils are the soul of aromatherapy candles. These oils are derived from various parts of plants, capturing the essence of their aromatic compounds. Choosing the right essential oils is key to achieving the desired therapeutic effects and fragrance. Lavender oil is popular for relaxation and stress relief, while eucalyptus oil is invigorating and ideal for colds and congestion. The number and combination of oils used dictate the complexity of the candle's fragrance.

Melting and Blending: Fusion of Elements

The wax is melted using a double boiler system, ensuring it reaches the desired temperature for optimal blending with the essential oils. Careful temperature management is crucial, as overheating can cause the essential oils to lose their potency. Once melted, the essential oils are added, and the mixture is stirred thoroughly to ensure an even distribution of the fragrance.

Pouring and Setting: Giving Shape to Fragrance

After blending, the wax mixture is poured into the chosen container or mold, where it solidifies into the desired shape. The wick is strategically placed to ensure even burning. As the candle cools and solidifies, it captures the essence of the essential oils, ready to release them upon lighting.

Choosing Essential Oils for Aromatherapy Candles: The Fragrance Palette

The selection of essential oils is an art in itself. Each essential oil possesses distinct properties and aromas, offering a wide palette for crafting the desired ambiance.

Lavender Essential Oil: The Classic Calm

Lavender, an iconic essential oil, is revered for its calming and relaxing properties. It's a go-to choice for those seeking a peaceful ambiance, making it perfect for bedrooms or spaces designated for rest and rejuvenation.

Citrus Essential Oils: The Energizing Zest

Citrus oils, like orange, lemon, and grapefruit, bring a burst of energy and vitality to any space. They uplift the mood and are excellent choices for common areas, providing an invigorating and refreshing ambiance.

Eucalyptus Essential Oil: The Respiratory Revive

Eucalyptus oil is widely known for its ability to clear the respiratory system and provide relief from congestion. A candle infused with eucalyptus oil is ideal for bathrooms or living areas, promoting a sense of freshness and cleanliness.

Peppermint Essential Oil: The Mind Refresher

Peppermint oil is famed for its ability to sharpen focus and alleviate mental fatigue. Having a candle with this invigorating scent in your workspace can enhance productivity and mental clarity.

The Art of Lighting Aromatherapy Candles: A Ritual of Tranquility

Lighting an aromatherapy candle is more than a mundane act; it's a ritual that ushers in tranquility and a sense of purpose. The process of igniting the wick and allowing the flame to dance as the scent subtly fills the room is therapeutic in itself.

Preparing the Space: Creating an Atmosphere

Before lighting the candle, set the ambiance. Dim the lights, play soft music, or engage in a brief meditation. Creating a serene environment amplifies the effects of the aromatherapy candle.

Lighting with Intent: Setting the Mood

As you light the candle, hold an intention in your mind—whether it's to relax, focus, or simply enjoy the moment. This intent infuses the candlelighting process with purpose and mindfulness.

Centering Yourself: Embracing the Calm

Take a moment to breathe and center yourself. Inhale the initial fragrances as they waft from the newly lit candle. Let the aroma encapsulate you and initiate a sense of tranquility.

Basking in the Glow: Moments of Reflection

Sit with the candle, observing the flickering flame and the gentle diffusion of fragrance. Use this time for self-reflection, meditation, or simply to be present in the moment, appreciating the subtle dance of light and scent.

Extinguishing with Gratitude: Closing the Ritual

When you're ready to conclude this sacred time, extinguish the candle with a sense of gratitude. Acknowledge the peace it brought and carry that energy forward into your day or evening.

Benefits of Aromatherapy Candles: Beyond the Fragrance

Aromatherapy candles offer a multitude of benefits beyond the pleasant scents they impart. These benefits are rooted in the therapeutic properties of the chosen essential oils.

Stress Reduction and Relaxation: Lavender's Embrace

Aromatherapy candles, especially those infused with lavender essential oil, have a calming effect on the mind and body. They can help reduce stress anxiety, and promote a restful night's sleep.

Respiratory Wellness: Eucalyptus and Peppermint's Aid

Candles infused with eucalyptus or peppermint essential oils can aid in respiratory wellness. The vapors released during burning can alleviate congestion and sinus issues.

Improved Focus and Concentration: The Peppermint Boost

Peppermint-scented candles are known to enhance focus and concentration. Lighting such a candle in a workspace can help in tasks that require mental clarity and attentiveness.

Mood Enhancement: Citrus and Beyond

Citrus-infused candles, with their refreshing and uplifting scents, can improve moods and create a positive atmosphere within a room. They are excellent choices for parties or gatherings.

Aromatherapy Candles: A Personal Touch to Atmosphere

Aromatherapy candles allow for personalization, enabling you to tailor the ambiance of your living spaces to your liking and needs. Whether you seek a calming retreat, an energizing workspace, or a cozy, romantic setting, the right aromatherapy candle can provide that and more.

Aromatherapy in Home Decor: The Fragrant Touch

Integrating aromatherapy candles into your home decor is an art. Place them strategically on coffee tables, shelves, or bathrooms to not only add fragrance but also enhance the aesthetic appeal of your space.

Gifting Aromatherapy: Sharing the Bliss

Aromatherapy candles make for thoughtful gifts. When selecting a candle for a friend or loved one, consider their preferences and the mood you wish to evoke, choosing an essential oil blend that resonates with them.

Safety Precautions: Nurturing the Flame

While aromatherapy candles bring immense joy, it's crucial to handle them with care and attention to safety.

Never Leave Unattended: The Watchful Eye

Ensure you extinguish the candle before leaving a room or going to sleep. Never leave a burning candle unattended, as it poses a fire hazard.

Trim the Wick: A Clean Burn

Before lighting the candle, trim the wick to approximately 1/4 inch. This ensures a clean, even burn and prevents excessive flame height.

Follow Instructions: Manufacturer's Wisdom

Adhere to the manufacturer's instructions regarding burning time and safety precautions. Different candles have varying burn times and safety guidelines.

Potpourri: Nature's Fragrant Bouquet

In the realm of enhancing ambiance through scent, potpourri stands as a time-honored tradition that has transcended centuries. A blend of dried flowers, herbs, and essential oils, potpourri is an artful way to bring the beauty of nature and its delightful fragrances into our homes. The term "potpourri" is derived from the French words "pot" (pot) and "pourrir" (to rot), signifying a mixture of substances allowed to mature in a pot to produce a fragrant concoction. This fragrant medley is more than just a pleasant aroma; it is a statement of elegance and a testament to the creative fusion of scents from the natural world.

The Artistry of Crafting Potpourri

Creating potpourri is an art that allows for personalization and creativity. The process begins with selecting a variety of dried flowers, herbs, and botanicals. Each component is chosen not only for its fragrance but also for its visual appeal, adding a touch of natural beauty to the blend. Some popular choices for potpourri ingredients include lavender, rose petals, citrus peels, eucalyptus leaves, cinnamon sticks, cloves, and dried berries.

Preparing the Ingredients

To start, you'll need to dry the chosen flowers and herbs thoroughly. This can be done by hanging them upside down in a cool, dark place. Once dried, gently remove the petals, leaves, and other plant parts from the stems. These components form the foundation of your potpourri.

Infusing with Essential Oils

After gathering the dried botanicals, it's time to infuse them with essential oils. Essential oils not only add fragrance but also help rejuvenate the dried components, giving them a burst of vitality. Choose essential oils that complement the natural scents of your chosen ingredients. Lavender essential oil, for example, pairs beautifully with dried lavender and rose petals.

Blending and Curing

Once the essential oils are added, gently mix the botanicals in a bowl, ensuring an even distribution of fragrance. Allow the mixture to cure in a closed container for a few weeks, allowing the oils to permeate the dried plants and infuse them with a rich, lasting scent. This curing process is essential to achieve a well-rounded and long-lasting potpourri.

Displaying Potpourri: The Visual and Fragrant Symphony

Potpourri is not only about its captivating aroma; it's also about visual appeal. The beauty of potpourri lies in its ability to serve as both a fragrant and decorative element in our living spaces. Displaying potpourri thoughtfully enhances the ambiance, creating a sensory symphony for anyone who enters the room.

Selecting Display Containers

The choice of containers for your potpourri is as important as the blend itself. It should resonate with the theme and aesthetics of the room. Decorative bowls, glass vases, ceramic dishes, or even mesh sachets can be used to hold and display the potpourri. The transparency of glass allows the natural colors and textures of the botanicals to be visible, adding to the visual appeal.

Strategically Placing Potpourri

The strategic placement of potpourri ensures its fragrance is evenly distributed throughout the room. Consider placing potpourri in high-traffic areas or near sources of natural airflow, like windows or vents. This allows the scent to disperse effectively, ensuring that the fragrance permeates the space.

Rotating and Refreshing

To maintain the potency of the fragrance, periodically rotate and refresh the potpourri. Gently fluff the mixture and add a few drops of the corresponding essential oils if needed. This simple step revitalizes the scent and extends the life of your potpourri.

Customizing Potpourri Blends: A Symphony of Scents

One of the joys of creating potpourri is the ability to customize the blend according to different preferences, seasons, or moods. The possibilities are endless, and each blend can evoke a unique ambiance within your living spaces.

Relaxation Blend

For a calming and relaxing ambiance, consider blending lavender, chamomile, and rose petals. Lavender provides a soothing aroma, chamomile induces a sense of tranquility, and rose petals add a touch of elegance to this blend. Place this in your bedroom or a quiet reading corner to unwind after a long day.

Energizing Blend

To infuse your living room or workspace with vitality and energy, create a blend using citrus peels, cloves, and cinnamon sticks. Citrus scents are known to be invigorating, while the warmth of cloves and cinnamon adds a comforting and uplifting touch, making it an ideal choice for communal areas where people gather.

Seasonal Variations

Adjust your potpourri blend according to the seasons to align with the changing natural scents and colors. In spring, incorporate blossoms and light floral scents. For autumn, use dried leaves, cinnamon, and pumpkin spice aromas. These seasonal variations not only reflect the changing times but also harmonize with the natural world.

Potpourri, the essence of nature captured in a fragrant bouquet, exemplifies the harmony between scent and aesthetics. It invites us to connect with the natural world within the confines of our homes, infusing our living spaces with an intoxicating blend of fragrances that rejuvenate our senses and calm our minds. Through the careful selection, preparation, and arrangement of dried botanicals and essential oils, we create an aromatic tapestry that adds depth and character to our surroundings. As we adorn our living spaces with this fragrant artistry, we invite the timeless beauty of nature into our homes, completing the holistic transformation into a sanctuary of well-being and harmony.

BOOK 7

DIY RECIPES AND APPLICATIONS

CHAPTER 1

MASSAGE BLENDS
FOR RELAXATION
AND PAIN RELIEF

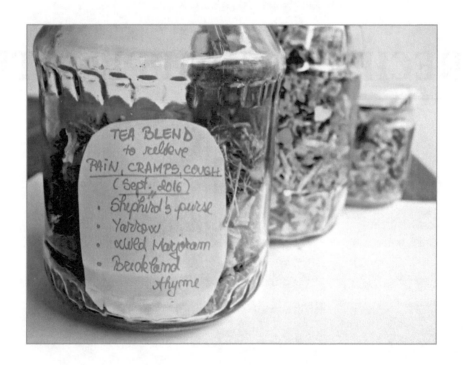

I n the realm of holistic wellness and self-care, the art of massage has proven to be a powerful and effective tool for relaxation and pain relief. Incorporating the use of natural and carefully blended massage oils can enhance the benefits of a massage, promoting relaxation, soothing sore muscles, and calming the mind. In this comprehensive guide, we will explore ten meticulously crafted massage oil recipes, each designed to serve specific purposes. The step-by-step instructions and detailed descriptions of the ingredients and their benefits will empower you to create your own personalized massage blends, ensuring a rejuvenating and healing massage experience.

RECIPE 1

LAVENDER AND CHAMOMILE RELAXATION BLEND

Ingredients:

- 30 ml carrier oil (such as sweet almond oil)
- 10 drops of lavender essential oil
- 5 drops of chamomile essential oil

Instructions:

1. Begin by choosing a clean glass bottle to store your blend.
2. Pour the carrier oil into the bottle, ensuring it's at least three-quarters full.
3. Add the lavender and chamomile essential oils to the carrier oil.
4. Close the bottle tightly and shake gently to blend the oils thoroughly.

1. Allow the blend to sit for 24 hours before using it to let the oils meld together.

Benefits:

- Lavender promotes relaxation and tranquility, reducing stress and anxiety.
- Chamomile calms the mind and aids in easing muscle tension, providing an overall soothing experience.

RECIPE 2

EUCALYPTUS AND PEPPERMINT MUSCLE RELIEF BLEND

Ingredients:

- 30 ml carrier oil (such as grapeseed oil)
- 10 drops eucalyptus essential oil
- 5 drops peppermint essential oil

Instructions:

2. Select a clean glass bottle to store your blend.
3. Pour the carrier oil into the bottle, filling it three-quarters of the way.
4. Add the eucalyptus and peppermint essential oils to the carrier oil.
5. Seal the bottle tightly and shake gently to combine the oils thoroughly.
6. Allow the blend to rest for 24 hours to achieve optimal fusion of the oils.

Benefits:

- Eucalyptus and peppermint oils have cooling properties that help relieve sore muscles and reduce inflammation.
- Eucalyptus oil promotes easier breathing and can be beneficial for respiratory issues.

RECIPE 3

FRANKINCENSE AND MYRRH RELAXATION BLEND

Ingredients:

- 30 ml carrier oil (such as jojoba oil)
- 10 drops of frankincense essential oil
- 5 drops of myrrh essential oil

Instructions:

1. Find a clean glass bottle for your blend.
2. Pour the carrier oil into the bottle, ensuring it fills about three-quarters of the bottle.
3. Add the frankincense and myrrh essential oils to the carrier oil.
4. Close the bottle tightly and gently shake to mix the oils thoroughly.
5. Allow the blend to rest for 24 hours before using.

Benefits:

- Frankincense and myrrh have anti-inflammatory properties, providing relaxation and aiding in relieving tension.
- The combined aroma of frankincense and myrrh promotes a sense of spiritual grounding and mental calmness.

RECIPE 4

CITRUS AND GINGER ENERGIZING BLEND

Ingredients:

- 30 ml carrier oil (such as coconut oil)
- 10 drops of orange essential oil
- 5 drops of lemon essential oil
- 3 drops of ginger essential oil

Instructions:

1. Use a clean glass bottle for your blend.
2. Pour the carrier oil into the bottle, filling it about three-quarters of the way.
3. Add the orange, lemon, and ginger essential oils to the carrier oil.
4. Seal the bottle tightly and shake gently to blend the oils thoroughly.
5. Allow the blend to sit for 24 hours before using.

Benefits:

- The citrus oils invigorate and uplift the spirit, promoting a sense of energy and vitality.
- Ginger essential oil aids in soothing sore muscles and provides a warming sensation, further enhancing relaxation.

RECIPE 5

ROSEMARY AND LAVENDER STRESS RELIEF BLEND

Ingredients:

- 30 ml carrier oil (such as apricot kernel oil)
- 10 drops rosemary essential oil
- 5 drops of lavender essential oil

Instructions:

1. Find a clean glass bottle for your blend.
2. Pour the carrier oil into the bottle, ensuring it's about three-quarters full.
3. Add the rosemary and lavender essential oils to the carrier oil.
4. Seal the bottle tightly and shake gently to mix the oils thoroughly.
5. Allow the blend to rest for 24 hours to achieve optimal fusion of the oils.

Benefits:

- Rosemary is known for its stress-relieving properties and can help alleviate headaches.
- Lavender promotes relaxation and can aid in reducing anxiety and emotional tension.

RECIPE 6

YLANG YLANG AND
BERGAMOT SENSUAL BLEND

Ingredients:

- 30 ml carrier oil (such as jojoba oil)
- 10 drops ylang-ylang essential oil
- 5 drops of bergamot essential oil

Instructions:

1. Select a clean glass bottle to store your blend.
2. Pour the carrier oil into the bottle, filling it three-quarters of the way.
3. Add the ylang-ylang and bergamot essential oils to the carrier oil.
4. Close the bottle tightly and shake gently to blend the oils thoroughly.
5. Allow the blend to rest for 24 hours before using.

Benefits:

- Ylang-ylang is known to enhance sensuality and promote a feeling of relaxation.
- Bergamot has mood-lifting properties and can help alleviate anxiety and stress.

RECIPE 7

CEDARWOOD AND PATCHOULI GROUNDING BLEND

Ingredients:

- 30 ml carrier oil (such as sweet almond oil)
- 10 drops of cedarwood essential oil
- 5 drops patchouli essential oil

Instructions:

1. Find a clean glass bottle for your blend.
2. Pour the carrier oil into the bottle, ensuring it's about three-quarters full.
3. Add the cedarwood and patchouli essential oils to the carrier oil.
4. Seal the bottle tightly and shake gently to mix the oils thoroughly.
5. Allow the blend to rest for 24 hours to achieve optimal fusion of the oils.

Benefits:

- Cedarwood is grounding and calming, promoting a sense of stability and balance.
- Patchouli has a relaxing and soothing effect on the mind and body, aiding in stress relief.

RECIPE 8

TEA TREE AND LAVENDER CLARIFYING BLEND

Ingredients:

- 30 ml carrier oil (such as grapeseed oil)
- 10 drops of tea tree essential oil
- 5 drops of lavender essential oil

Instructions:

1. Use a clean glass bottle for your blend.
2. Pour the carrier oil into the bottle, filling it about three-quarters of the way.
3. Add the tea tree and lavender essential oils to the carrier oil.
4. Seal the bottle tightly and shake gently to combine the oils thoroughly.
5. Allow the blend to rest for 24 hours before using.

Benefits:

- Tea tree oil has antibacterial properties, making this blend beneficial for cleansing and clarifying the skin.
- Lavender complements tea trees by providing a calming and soothing effect.

RECIPE 9

PEPPERMINT AND LAVENDER HEADACHE RELIEF BLEND

Ingredients:

- 30 ml carrier oil (such as coconut oil)
- 10 drops peppermint essential oil
- 5 drops of lavender essential oil

Instructions:

1. Select a clean glass bottle to store your blend.
2. Pour the carrier oil into the bottle, ensuring it fills about three-quarters of the bottle.
3. Add the peppermint and lavender essential oils to the carrier oil.
4. Close the bottle tightly and shake gently to blend the oils thoroughly.
5. Allow the blend to sit for 24 hours before using.

Benefits:

- Peppermint oil provides a cooling sensation that can alleviate headaches and migraines.
- Lavender contributes to relaxation and aids in reducing tension, enhancing the blend's headache-relieving properties.

RECIPE 10

GINGER AND TURMERIC ANTI-INFLAMMATORY BLEND

Ingredients:

- 30 ml carrier oil (such as apricot kernel oil)
- 10 drops of ginger essential oil
- 5 drops turmeric essential oil

Instructions:

1. Find a clean glass bottle for your blend.
2. Pour the carrier oil into the bottle, ensuring it's about three-quarters full.
3. Add the ginger and turmeric essential oils to the carrier oil.
4. Seal the bottle tightly and shake gently to mix the oils thoroughly.
5. Allow the blend to rest for 24 hours before using.

Benefits:

- Ginger and turmeric have potent anti-inflammatory properties, making this blend ideal for sore muscles and joint pain.
- The warming effect of ginger further enhances muscle relaxation and soothing.

The art of massage, combined with the power of carefully crafted massage oil blends, holds the key to a profoundly relaxing and rejuvenating experience. These ten DIY massage oil recipes offer a diverse range of benefits, from relaxation and stress relief to pain management and skin cleansing. By creating these blends and incorporating them into your self-care routine, you can harness the therapeutic properties of essential oils to enhance your overall well-being. Remember to always choose high-quality, pure essential oils and carrier oils to ensure the efficacy and safety of your massage blends. Enjoy the soothing effects of these natural creations as you embark on a journey of self-care and holistic healing.

CHAPTER 2

BATH AND BODY PRODUCTS

(BATH SALTS, SHOWER GELS, LOTIONS)

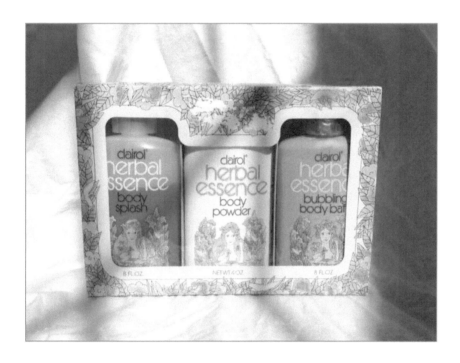

Creating DIY bath and body products can be a delightful and fulfilling venture, offering not only the joy of a personal touch but also the benefit of knowing exactly what goes into the products you use on your skin. In this section, we will delve into the realm of DIY bath and body products, particularly focusing on bath salts, shower gels, and lotions. These simple yet luxurious concoctions can elevate your self-care routine and contribute to a healthier, more radiant you. We will be discussing ten unique and delightful recipes for each of these products, providing step-by-step guides and detailing the benefits they offer.

BATH SALTS RECIPES

1

LAVENDER AND
EPSOM SALT SOAK

Ingredients:

- 1 cup Epsom salt
- 1/2 cup baking soda
- 10-15 drops of lavender essential oil
- Dried lavender buds (optional)

Instructions:

1. Mix Epsom salt and baking soda in a bowl.
2. Add the lavender essential oil and mix thoroughly.
3. Transfer the mixture into an airtight container and add dried lavender buds if desired.
4. To use, add a generous amount to your bath and soak for at least 20 minutes.

Benefits:

- Epsom salt helps soothe sore muscles and reduce stress.
- Lavender essential oil promotes relaxation and a calm mind.

2

CITRUS ZEST BATH SALT

Ingredients:

- 1 cup Epsom salt
- Zest of 1 lemon and 1 orange
- 10-15 drops of lemon essential oil
- 10-15 drops of sweet orange essential oil

Instructions:

1. Combine Epsom salt and citrus zest in a mixing bowl.
2. Add the lemon and sweet orange essential oils and mix thoroughly.
3. Store in an airtight container.
4. Use a few spoonfuls in your bath for a refreshing soak.

Benefits:

- Citrus oils invigorate and refresh the senses.
- Epsom salt aids in detoxifying the body and improving circulation.

3

ROSE PETAL AND HIMALAYAN SALT BATH

Ingredients:

- 1 cup Himalayan salt
- 1/2 cup dried rose petals
- 10-15 drops of rose essential oil

Instructions:

1. Combine Himalayan salt and dried rose petals in a bowl.
2. Add the rose essential oil and mix well.
3. Transfer to an airtight container.
4. Use a handful in your bath for a luxurious and aromatic soak.

Benefits:

- Himalayan salt helps in balancing the body's pH and mineral levels.
- Rose essential oil promotes relaxation and rejuvenation.

4

PEPPERMINT AND GREEN TEA BATH SALT

Ingredients:

- 1 cup Epsom salt
- 2-3 peppermint tea bags
- 10-15 drops of peppermint essential oil
- 1 tablespoon green tea leaves

Instructions:

1. Cut open the tea bags and mix the green tea leaves with Epsom salt.
2. Add the peppermint essential oil and blend well.
3. Transfer to an airtight container.
4. Use a few tablespoons in your bath for a refreshing and revitalizing experience.

Benefits:

- Peppermint promotes mental clarity and alleviates fatigue.
- Green tea leaves offer antioxidants and detoxifying properties.

5

CHAMOMILE AND OATMEAL BATH SOAK

Ingredients:

- 1 cup Epsom salt
- 1/2 cup colloidal oatmeal
- 10-15 drops of chamomile essential oil

Instructions:

1. Mix Epsom salt and colloidal oatmeal in a bowl.
2. Add the chamomile essential oil and blend thoroughly.
3. Store in an airtight container.
4. Use a scoop in your bath for a soothing and gentle soak.

Benefits:

- Chamomile essential oil calms the skin and relaxes the body.
- Colloidal oatmeal soothes irritated skin and provides moisture.

SHOWER GEL RECIPES

1

REFRESHING CITRUS
SHOWER GEL

Ingredients:

- 1/2 cup liquid castile soap
- 1/4 cup aloe vera gel
- 1/4 cup sweet almond oil
- 10-15 drops of lemon essential oil
- 10-15 drops of sweet orange essential oil

Instructions:

1. In a mixing bowl, combine liquid castile soap, aloe vera gel, and sweet almond oil.
2. Add lemon and sweet orange essential oils and mix thoroughly.
3. Pour into a clean, empty shower gel bottle.
4. Use as you would any commercial shower gel.

Benefits:

- Aloe vera soothes and hydrates the skin.
- Citrus essential oils invigorate and refresh your senses.

2

CALMING LAVENDER AND CHAMOMILE SHOWER GEL

Ingredients:

- 1/2 cup liquid castile soap
- 1/4 cup aloe vera gel
- 1/4 cup jojoba oil
- 10-15 drops of lavender essential oil
- 10-15 drops of chamomile essential oil

Instructions:

1. Mix liquid castile soap, aloe vera gel, and jojoba oil in a bowl.
2. Add lavender and chamomile essential oils and blend well.
3. Transfer to a clean, empty shower gel bottle.
4. Enjoy a soothing and calming shower experience.

Benefits:

- Jojoba oil moisturizes and balances skin.
- Lavender and chamomile essential oils promote relaxation.

3

ENERGIZING MINTY SHOWER GEL

Ingredients:

- 1/2 cup liquid castile soap
- 1/4 cup aloe vera gel
- 1/4 cup grapeseed oil
- 10-15 drops of peppermint essential oil
- 10-15 drops of eucalyptus essential oil

Instructions:

1. Combine liquid castile soap, aloe vera gel, and grapeseed oil in a bowl.
2. Add peppermint and eucalyptus essential oils and mix thoroughly.
3. Pour into a clean, empty shower gel bottle.
4. Enjoy the refreshing and energizing scent during your shower.

Benefits:

- Peppermint and eucalyptus essential oils awaken and invigorate the senses.
- Grapeseed oil nourishes the skin with vitamins and antioxidants.

4

HONEY AND OATMEAL SHOWER GEL

Ingredients:

- 1/2 cup liquid castile soap
- 1/4 cup aloe vera gel
- 1/4 cup honey
- 2 tablespoons colloidal oatmeal

Instructions:

1. In a bowl, mix liquid castile soap, aloe vera gel, and honey.
2. Add colloidal oatmeal and blend until smooth.
3. Transfer to a clean, empty shower gel bottle.
4. Use it for a soothing and hydrating shower experience.

Benefits:

- Honey has antibacterial properties and helps retain moisture.
- Colloidal oatmeal soothes and nourishes the skin.

5

TEA TREE AND LAVENDER ANTISEPTIC SHOWER GEL

Ingredients:

- 1/2 cup liquid castile soap
- 1/4 cup aloe vera gel
- 1/4 cup jojoba oil
- 10-15 drops of tea tree essential oil
- 10-15 drops of lavender essential oil

Instructions:

1. Mix liquid castile soap, aloe vera gel, and jojoba oil in a bowl.
2. Add tea tree and lavender essential oils and blend well.
3. Pour into a clean, empty shower gel bottle.
4. Enjoy the antiseptic and calming properties of this shower gel.

Benefits:

- Tea tree essential oil has antibacterial and antifungal properties.
- Jojoba oil moisturizes and balances the skin.

LOTIONS RECIPES

1

NOURISHING SHEA BUTTER LOTION

Ingredients:

- 1/2 cup shea butter
- 1/4 cup coconut oil
- 1/4 cup sweet almond oil
- 10-15 drops of your favorite essential oil (e.g., lavender, rose)

Instructions:

1. In a double boiler, melt shea butter, coconut oil, and sweet almond oil until fully liquid.
2. Allow the mixture to cool slightly before adding the essential oil.
3. Transfer to a clean, airtight container and let it solidify into a creamy lotion.
4. Apply to your skin for a deeply moisturizing and nourishing experience.

Benefits:

- Shea butter and coconut oil deeply moisturize and soften the skin.
- Sweet almond oil provides essential fatty acids and vitamins.

2

COOLING ALOE VERA
AND MINT LOTION

Ingredients:

- 1/2 cup aloe vera gel
- 1/4 cup coconut oil
- 1/4 cup jojoba oil
- 10-15 drops of peppermint essential oil

Instructions:

1. In a mixing bowl, combine aloe vera gel, coconut oil, and jojoba oil.
2. Add peppermint essential oil and mix until well incorporated.
3. Transfer to a clean, airtight container.
4. Store in the refrigerator for a cooling sensation when applied.

Benefits:

- Aloe vera soothes and hydrates the skin.
- Peppermint essential oil provides a refreshing and cooling effect.

3

REJUVENATING GREEN TEA AND CUCUMBER LOTION

Ingredients:

- 1/2 cup green tea-infused water (cooled)
- 1/4 cup shea butter
- 1/4 cup grapeseed oil
- 10-15 drops of cucumber essential oil

Instructions:

1. Infuse green tea in water and let it cool.
2. In a double boiler, melt shea butter and grapeseed oil until fully liquid.
3. Allow the mixture to cool slightly before adding the cucumber essential oil and green tea.
4. Transfer to a clean, airtight container and let it solidify into a lotion.

Benefits:

- Green tea offers antioxidants and anti-aging properties.
- Cucumber essential oil refreshes and rejuvenates the skin.

4

MOISTURIZING HONEY AND ALMOND OIL LOTION

Ingredients:

- 1/2 cup almond oil
- 1/4 cup coconut oil
- 1/4 cup honey

Instructions:

1. In a mixing bowl, combine almond oil, coconut oil, and honey.
2. Mix well until the ingredients are thoroughly combined.
3. Transfer to a clean, airtight container.
4. Apply to your skin for a moisturizing and hydrating experience.

Benefits:

- Almond oil nourishes and softens the skin.
- Honey provides antibacterial and moisturizing properties.

5

LAVENDER AND CHAMOMILE CALMING LOTION

Ingredients:

- 1/2 cup almond oil
- 1/4 cup shea butter
- 1/4 cup cocoa butter
- 10-15 drops of lavender essential oil
- 10-15 drops of chamomile essential oil

Instructions:

1. In a double boiler, melt almond oil, shea butter, and cocoa butter until fully liquid.
2. Allow the mixture to cool slightly before adding the lavender and chamomile essential oils.
3. Transfer to a clean, airtight container and let it solidify into a creamy lotion.
4. Apply to your skin for a calming and soothing experience.

Benefits:

- Lavender and chamomile essential oils promote relaxation and reduce stress.
- Shea butter and cocoa butter deeply moisturize and nourish the skin.

CHAPTER 3
NATURAL PERFUMES
AND FRAGRANCES

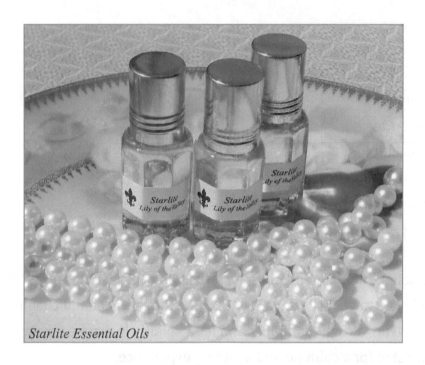

Starlite Essential Oils

n a world increasingly embracing natural and eco-friendly alternatives, the realm of personal care products is no exception. One of the fascinating aspects of this movement is the rise of DIY (Do-It-Yourself) beauty products, particularly natural perfumes and fragrances. Crafting your own fragrances not only allows for customization according to personal preferences but also guarantees the use of safe, natural ingredients. Book 7 delves into this enticing world of DIY recipes and applications, focusing on creating exquisite natural perfumes and fragrances. This chapter presents ten detailed DIY perfume recipes, offering a step-by-step guide to their creation and discussing the numerous benefits of using natural ingredients in your perfumes.

I

LAVENDER DREAMS PERFUME

Lavender has long been admired for its calming and relaxing properties. Creating a perfume using lavender can provide a soothing fragrance ideal for any occasion.

Ingredients:

- Lavender essential oil
- Distilled water
- Jojoba oil

Steps:

1. Begin by choosing a small glass perfume bottle as your container.
2. Add 20-25 drops of lavender essential oil into the bottle, depending on your preference for scent intensity.
3. Pour distilled water into the bottle, filling it almost to the top.
4. Add 1-2 teaspoons of jojoba oil to the mix, which will help bind the essential oil and water.
5. Close the bottle and shake gently to combine all the ingredients.
6. Allow the perfume to sit for a day to let the scents meld.
7. Apply by dabbing a small amount on your pulse points.

Benefits:

- Lavender has a calming effect, making this perfume perfect for reducing stress and anxiety.
- It may also aid in promoting better sleep and relieving headaches.

II

CITRUS BURST PERFUME

Citrus scents are known for their invigorating and refreshing qualities, making them a popular choice for perfumes. This DIY citrus perfume will awaken your senses and energize your day.

Ingredients:

- Sweet orange essential oil
- Lemon essential oil
- Grapefruit essential oil
- Vodka (as a base)

Steps:

1. In a glass perfume bottle, combine 10 drops of sweet orange essential oil, 7 drops of lemon essential oil, and 5 drops of grapefruit essential oil.
2. Fill the rest of the bottle with vodka, leaving a little space at the top.
3. Close the bottle and shake gently to mix the oils and vodka.
4. Allow the perfume to sit for 24-48 hours, allowing the scents to meld and blend.
5. Apply sparingly to your pulse points and enjoy the refreshing fragrance.

Benefits:

- Citrus scents are known to boost mood and energy levels, making this perfume ideal for a quick pick-me-up.
- The natural oils in this perfume can also have antimicrobial properties, potentially providing a mild antiseptic effect.

III

ROSE GARDEN PERFUME

Roses have long been associated with beauty and romance, making them a timeless choice for fragrances. Creating a rose-scented perfume at home allows you to capture the essence of a blooming rose garden.

Ingredients:

- Rose essential oil
- Jojoba oil
- Distilled water

Steps:

1. Select a glass perfume bottle for your mixture.
2. Add 20-25 drops of rose essential oil to the bottle.
3. Fill the bottle with distilled water, leaving a little space at the top.
4. Add 1-2 teaspoons of jojoba oil to help combine the essential oil with the water.
5. Close the bottle and shake gently to mix the ingredients.
6. Allow the perfume to sit for a day to let the scents blend.
7. Apply a small amount to your pulse points for a delicate, rosy fragrance.

Benefits:

- Rose essential oil is believed to have mood-enhancing and stress-reducing properties, making this perfume perfect for relaxation and tranquility.
- The floral scent of roses can also act as a natural mood lifter, promoting a sense of well-being.

IV

WOODSY ELEGANCE PERFUME

For those who appreciate the rustic charm of the outdoors, a woody perfume can bring the essence of nature to their daily routine. This DIY perfume embodies the scent of a serene forest.

Ingredients:

- Cedarwood essential oil
- Sandalwood essential oil
- Jojoba oil

Steps:

1. Select a glass perfume bottle to hold your mixture.
2. Add 15 drops of cedarwood essential oil and 10 drops of sandalwood essential oil to the bottle.
3. Top off the bottle with jojoba oil, leaving a small space at the top.
4. Close the bottle and gently shake to blend the oils and jojoba.
5. Allow the perfume to sit for a day to let the fragrances harmonize.
6. Apply sparingly to your pulse points and relish the woody aroma.

Benefits:

- Cedarwood and sandalwood scents are associated with grounding and calming effects, making this perfume ideal for finding balance and centering oneself.
- The natural woodsy scent can evoke a sense of nature, promoting relaxation and connection with the outdoors.

V

JASMINE NIGHTS PERFUME

Jasmine is renowned for its sweet, floral fragrance and is often used in perfumery. Capturing the essence of jasmine in a DIY perfume allows you to enjoy its exquisite scent throughout the day.

Ingredients:

- Jasmine essential oil
- Fractionated coconut oil
- Distilled water

Steps:

1. Choose a glass perfume bottle to mix your perfume.
2. Add 20-25 drops of jasmine essential oil to the bottle.
3. Fill the bottle with distilled water, leaving some space at the top.
4. Pour in a small amount of fractionated coconut oil to help blend the essential oil and water.
5. Close the bottle and shake gently to combine all the ingredients.
6. Allow the perfume to sit for a day to allow the scents to merge.
7. Apply a small amount to your pulse points and enjoy the delicate floral aroma.

Benefits:

- Jasmine essential oil is believed to have mood-enhancing properties and may help reduce feelings of anxiety and stress.
- The sweet, floral scent of jasmine can also act as a natural aphrodisiac, enhancing feelings of love and intimacy.

VI

MINTY FRESH PERFUME

Mint is well-known for its invigorating and revitalizing qualities. This DIY perfume harnesses the crisp, cool scent of mint, providing a refreshing fragrance.

Ingredients:

- Peppermint essential oil
- Spearmint essential oil
- Fractionated coconut oil

Steps:

1. Select a glass perfume bottle to hold your mixture.
2. Combine 15 drops of peppermint essential oil and 10 drops of spearmint essential oil in the bottle.
3. Add a small amount of fractionated coconut oil to the bottle.
4. Close the bottle and gently shake to mix the oils and coconut oil.
5. Allow the perfume to sit for a day to let the scents blend.
6. Apply a small amount to your pulse points and experience the refreshing, minty aroma.

Benefits:

- Minty scents are known to boost alertness and focus, making this perfume ideal for a quick energy boost during the day.
- The invigorating scent of mint can also help alleviate headaches and migraines.

VII

FLORAL HARMONY PERFUME

A blend of various floral scents can create a harmonious and elegant perfume. This DIY floral perfume combines the best of floral essences, providing a captivating aroma.

Ingredients:

- Lavender essential oil
- Rose essential oil
- Ylang-ylang essential oil
- Jojoba oil
- Distilled water

Steps:

1. Choose a glass perfume bottle for your mixture.
2. Combine 10 drops of lavender essential oil, 10 drops of rose essential oil, and 5 drops of ylang-ylang essential oil in the bottle.
3. Fill the bottle with distilled water, leaving a little space at the top.
4. Add 1-2 teaspoons of jojoba oil to help blend the oils and water.
5. Close the bottle and shake gently to combine all the ingredients.
6. Allow the perfume to sit for a day to let the scents meld and create a balanced fragrance.
7. Apply a small amount to your pulse points and enjoy the delicate floral blend.

Benefits:

- The combination of different floral scents can evoke a sense of tranquility and relaxation, promoting a calm and peaceful state of mind.

- Floral fragrances are often associated with happiness and a positive outlook, enhancing one's mood and well-being.

VIII

SPICED VANILLA PERFUME

Vanilla is a classic scent loved by many for its sweet and comforting aroma. Adding a hint of spice elevates the perfume, creating a warm and inviting fragrance.

Ingredients:

- Vanilla essential oil or vanilla extract
- Cinnamon essential oil
- Jojoba oil

Steps:

1. Choose a glass perfume bottle to hold your mixture.
2. Add 15-20 drops of vanilla essential oil or a small amount of vanilla extract to the bottle.
3. Incorporate 5-10 drops of cinnamon essential oil into the mixture.
4. Top off the bottle with jojoba oil, leaving a small space at the top.
5. Close the bottle and gently shake to blend the oils and jojoba.
6. Allow the perfume to sit for a day to let the scents blend and create a delightful fragrance.
7. Apply a small amount to your pulse points and enjoy the comforting, spiced vanilla aroma.

Benefits:

- Vanilla has a calming effect, promoting relaxation and reducing stress and anxiety.
- Cinnamon is believed to have invigorating and stimulating properties, potentially enhancing alertness and concentration.

IX

EARTHY PATCHOULI PERFUME

Patchouli is a unique and distinct scent often associated with earthiness and grounding. Creating a perfume using patchouli allows you to capture its rich, aromatic essence.

Ingredients:

- Patchouli essential oil
- Fractionated coconut oil

Steps:

1. Choose a glass perfume bottle for your mixture.
2. Add 20-25 drops of patchouli essential oil to the bottle.
3. Top off the bottle with fractionated coconut oil, leaving a small space at the top.
4. Close the bottle and gently shake to blend the oils and coconut oil.
5. Allow the perfume to sit for a day to let the scents meld and create a harmonious fragrance.
6. Apply a small amount to your pulse points and relish the earthy, grounding aroma.

Benefits:

- Patchouli is often associated with grounding and balancing effects, making this perfume ideal for finding inner peace and stability.
- The earthy scent of patchouli can also have a relaxing and calming effect on the mind.

X

FRESH AND ZESTY PERFUME

Combining fresh and zesty scents creates a lively and invigorating perfume that's perfect for a burst of energy throughout the day. This DIY perfume combines citrus and herbal elements for a vibrant fragrance.

Ingredients:

- Lime essential oil
- Bergamot essential oil
- Rosemary essential oil
- Jojoba oil

Steps:

1. Select a glass perfume bottle for your mixture.
2. Add 10 drops of lime essential oil, 10 drops of bergamot essential oil, and 5 drops of rosemary essential oil to the bottle.
3. Fill the bottle with jojoba oil, leaving a little space at the top.
4. Close the bottle and gently shake to combine all the oils and jojoba.
5. Allow the perfume to sit for a day to let the scents blend and create a fresh, zesty fragrance.
6. Apply a small amount to your pulse points and enjoy the lively, invigorating aroma.

Benefits:

- The fresh and zesty scents can uplift and energize, providing a mood-boosting effect throughout the day.
- Rosemary is believed to have cognitive-enhancing properties, potentially improving concentration and memory.

Creating your own natural perfumes and fragrances using DIY recipes allows you to personalize your scents while ensuring the use of safe, natural ingredients. Each recipe presented in this chapter offers a unique blend of scents and benefits, allowing you to explore and experiment with various fragrances. From the calming lavender to the invigorating citrus burst, these perfumes cater to different moods and occasions, enhancing your overall well-being and leaving a lasting, natural impression. Dive into the world of DIY perfumery, and let your creativity flow as you craft fragrances that reflect your personality and preferences.

CHAPTER 4

HOME SPA
TREATMENTS

(FACIAL MASKS, BODY SCRUBS,
HAIR TREATMENTS)

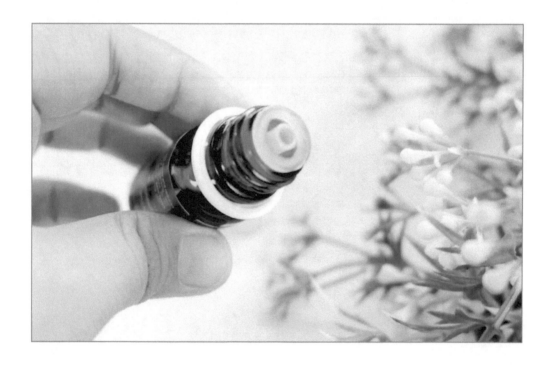

In today's fast-paced world, finding time to visit a spa for relaxation and self-care can be challenging. However, self-pampering doesn't have to be compromised. With the right knowledge and simple ingredients from your pantry, you can create your own spa-like experience at home. This book, Book 7: DIY Recipes and Applications, delves into the art of creating rejuvenating and indulgent home spa treatments, including facial masks, body scrubs, and hair treatments. We will provide ten comprehensive recipes with step-by-step guides for each, unveiling the secrets of home spa treatments and the various benefits they offer for your skin, body, and hair.

1

LAVENDER AND HONEY RELAXING FACIAL MASK

Ingredients:

- 2 tablespoons of lavender buds
- 1 tablespoon of raw honey
- 1 tablespoon of plain yogurt

Instructions:

1. Grind the lavender buds to a fine powder.
2. Mix the lavender powder, honey, and yogurt in a bowl to form a smooth paste.
3. Apply the mixture evenly on your face and neck.
4. Leave it on for 15-20 minutes.
5. Rinse off with warm water.

Benefits:

- Lavender calms the skin and senses, promoting relaxation.
- Honey is a natural humectant, moisturizing and softening the skin.
- Yogurt provides a gentle exfoliation and nourishes the skin.

2

COFFEE AND COCONUT OIL BODY SCRUB

Ingredients:

- 1/2 cup of ground coffee
- 1/4 cup of coconut oil
- 1/4 cup of brown sugar

Instructions:

1. Mix all the ingredients in a bowl to create a grainy paste.
2. Apply the scrub to damp skin, gently massaging in circular motions.
3. Focus on rough areas like elbows, knees, and feet.
4. Rinse off with warm water and pat dry.

Benefits

- Coffee exfoliates, stimulating circulation and reducing cellulite.
- Coconut oil moisturizes and nourishes the skin.
- Brown sugar provides additional exfoliation and a sweet scent.

4

AVOCADO AND
BANANA HAIR MASK

Ingredients:

- 1 ripe avocado
- 1 ripe banana
- 2 tablespoons of olive oil

Instructions:

1. Mash the avocado and banana in a bowl until smooth.
2. Add olive oil and mix well to form a creamy paste.
3. Apply the mask to damp hair, starting from the roots to the tips.
4. Cover your hair with a shower cap and leave it on for 30-45 minutes.
5. Rinse thoroughly and shampoo as usual.

Benefits:

- Avocado nourishes and adds shine to the hair.
- Banana helps prevent hair breakage and split ends.
- Olive oil provides deep conditioning and moisturizes the scalp.

5

TURMERIC AND CHICKPEA FLOUR BRIGHTENING FACE MASK

Ingredients

- 1 tablespoon of turmeric powder
- 2 tablespoons of chickpea flour
- Rosewater (as needed)

Instructions:

1. Mix turmeric powder and chickpea flour in a bowl.
2. Slowly add rosewater to make a smooth paste.
3. Apply the mask to your face and neck, avoiding the eye area.
4. Let it dry for 15-20 minutes.
5. Gently scrub off the mask using warm water.

Benefits:

- Turmeric brightens and evens out the skin tone.
- Chickpea flour exfoliates and removes dead skin cells.
- Rosewater soothes and refreshes the skin.

6

OATMEAL AND HONEY SOOTHING BATH SOAK

Ingredients:

- 1 cup of oats
- 1/4 cup of honey
- Lavender essential oil (a few drops)

Instructions:

1. Grind the oats to a fine powder using a blender.
2. Mix the powdered oats, honey, and lavender oil in a bowl.
3. Add the mixture to your bathwater while it's running.
4. Soak in the bath for 20-30 minutes.

Benefits:

- Oats soothe and calm irritated skin.
- Honey moisturizes and softens the skin.
- Lavender oil promotes relaxation and reduces stress.

7

LEMON AND SUGAR LIP SCRUB

Ingredients:

- 1 tablespoon of white sugar
- 1 tablespoon of brown sugar
- 1/2 tablespoon of coconut oil
- 1/2 teaspoon of lemon juice

Instructions:

1. Mix all the ingredients in a small bowl to create a grainy paste.
2. Gently massage the scrub onto your lips in circular motions for a minute.
3. Rinse off with warm water and pat dry.

Benefits:

- Sugar exfoliates and removes dead skin from the lips.
- Coconut oil moisturizes and nourishes the lips.
- Lemon juice brightens and refreshes the lips.

8

GREEN TEA AND ALOE VERA COOLING FACE MIST

Ingredients:

- 1 green tea bag
- 1/4 cup of aloe vera juice
- 1/4 cup of distilled water

Instructions:

1. Brew the green tea bag in hot water and let it cool.
2. Mix the brewed green tea, aloe vera juice, and distilled water in a spray bottle.
3. Shake well and store in the refrigerator.
4. Spray on your face for a refreshing and cooling effect.

Benefits:

- Green tea is rich in antioxidants, promoting healthy and rejuvenated skin.
- Aloe vera soothes and hydrates the skin.
- The mist revitalizes and cools the skin, especially on a hot day.

9

ROSEMARY AND OLIVE OIL SCALP MASSAGE

Ingredients:

- 2 tablespoons of fresh rosemary leaves
- 1/4 cup of olive oil

Instructions:

1. Heat the olive oil in a small pan and add the rosemary leaves.
2. Let it simmer for a few minutes until the oil is infused with the rosemary fragrance.
3. Allow the oil to cool down to a warm temperature.
4. Massage the oil into your scalp using gentle circular motions for 10-15 minutes.
5. Leave it on for an additional 30 minutes before shampooing.

Benefits:

- Rosemary stimulates hair growth and improves circulation in the scalp.
- Olive oil nourishes and strengthens the hair, leaving it soft and shiny.

10

CUCUMBER AND MINT REFRESHING EYE MASK

Ingredients:

- 1/2 cucumber
- A handful of fresh mint leaves

Instructions:

1. Blend the cucumber and mint leaves to form a smooth paste.
2. Apply the paste around your eyes and on your eyelids.
3. Lie down and leave it on for 15-20 minutes.
4. Gently wipe off the mask with a damp cotton pad.

Benefits:

- Cucumber reduces puffiness and dark circles around the eyes.
- Mint refreshes and soothes the delicate skin around the eyes.

11

HONEY AND ALOE VERA HEALING FACE MASK

Ingredients:

- 1 tablespoon of raw honey
- 2 tablespoons of aloe vera gel

Instructions:

1. Mix the honey and aloe vera gel in a bowl until well combined.
2. Apply the mask to your face and neck, avoiding the eye area.
3. Let it sit for 20-25 minutes.
4. Rinse off with warm water.

Benefits:

- Honey has antibacterial properties, keeping the skin clear and acne-free.
- Aloe vera soothes and heals the skin, reducing inflammation.

Creating your own spa treatments at home not only allows for a pampering experience but also provides the opportunity to use natural and wholesome ingredients that benefit your skin, body, and hair. The recipes provided in this book, with step-by-step guides and detailed benefits, empower you to indulge in self-care and attain a rejuvenated and radiant appearance without leaving the comfort of your home. Experiment with these recipes, tailor them to your preferences and embrace the delightful journey of self-pampering and well-being.

FAQ

1. What are essential oils?

Essential oils are highly concentrated, aromatic compounds extracted from various parts of plants. These oils capture the plant's essence and are renowned for their therapeutic properties and distinct scents.

2. How does aromatherapy work?

Aromatherapy is a holistic healing practice that uses essential oils to promote physical, mental, and emotional well-being. Inhaling or applying essential oils can affect the limbic system in the brain, influencing emotions, stress levels, and overall health.

3. What is the history of aromatherapy?

Aromatherapy has ancient origins, dating back thousands of years across different cultures. It was used for medicinal, spiritual, and cosmetic purposes, with the practice evolving and gaining popularity over time.

4. What are the extraction methods for essential oils?

Essential oils are extracted through various methods, including steam distillation, cold pressing, solvent extraction, and CO_2 extraction. Each method has its own set of benefits and is suitable for different types of plant materials.

5. Are there any safety guidelines for using essential oils?

Yes, essential oils are potent and should be used with caution. Dilution, skin patch tests, avoiding ingestion of certain oils, and consulting a professional before use, especially during pregnancy or for children, are important safety precautions.

6. How can essential oils boost immunity?

Certain essential oils possess immune-boosting properties that can support the immune system when inhaled or applied topically. These oils can aid in preventing illnesses and promoting overall health.

7. Can essential oils help with respiratory health?

Yes, specific essential oils can help relieve congestion, support sinus health, and improve respiratory function when used in inhalation techniques or diffusers.

8. Are essential oils effective for natural pain relief?

Yes, anti-inflammatory essential oils and topical applications can provide natural pain relief for various conditions like muscle soreness, headaches, or joint pain.

9. Can essential oils aid in digestive health?

Essential oils with digestive properties can be used in massage techniques to ease digestive discomfort and promote a healthy digestive system.

10. How can essential oils assist in stress management and relaxation?

Calming essential oils, when diffused or applied, can reduce stress levels and induce relaxation, supporting overall mental well-being.

11. Can essential oils improve mood?

Yes, uplifting essential oils and aromatherapy blends can positively impact mood and emotional states, promoting a more cheerful and balanced outlook.

12. Do essential oils help with focus and concentration?

Stimulating essential oils can enhance focus and concentration, making them valuable for work or study environments.

13. Are there essential oils that support better sleep?

Indeed, soothing essential oils can aid in promoting better sleep when used in bedtime rituals or diffused in the sleeping environment.

14. How can essential oils enhance skincare and beauty routines?

Essential oils can be incorporated into facial care, body care, hair care, and natural perfumes to improve the health and appearance of the skin, body, and hair.

15. Can essential oils be used for natural cleaning?

Yes, essential oils can be used for natural cleaning, offering antimicrobial properties and a pleasant scent for homemade cleaning solutions.

ESSENTIAL OILS FOR NATURAL CLEANING AND HOME CARE

Essential Oils for Cleaning

Cleaning is an essential aspect of maintaining a healthy and pleasant living environment. However, with concerns about the environmental and health impacts of conventional cleaning products, there's a growing interest in finding natural and eco-friendly alternatives. Essential oils have emerged as a popular choice, offering a range of properties that make them effective for cleaning various surfaces in a natural and safe manner.

Essential Oils for Surface Cleaning

Surface cleaning is a regular household task that involves disinfecting and removing dirt and grime from different surfaces like countertops, floors, windows, and more. Essential oils can be powerful tools in achieving a sparkling and clean home, replacing harsh chemicals with a natural approach.

Lemon Essential Oil

Lemon essential oil, derived from the peel of lemons through cold pressing, is a versatile and widely used essential oil in cleaning. It is renowned for its potent grease-cutting abilities and its fresh, citrusy scent. The high limonene content in lemon oil provides powerful cleaning properties, making it an excellent choice for tackling kitchen surfaces.

When used for surface cleaning, lemon essential oil can effectively remove grease, grime, and stains. It can be utilized to clean countertops, cutting boards, sinks, and other kitchen surfaces. Here's a simple DIY all-purpose cleaner using lemon essential oil:

Lemon All-Purpose Cleaner Recipe:

- 1 cup water
- 1/2 cup white vinegar
- 15-20 drops of lemon essential oil

Combine these ingredients in a spray bottle and shake well before use. Spray the mixture onto surfaces and wipe clean with a cloth. The lemon essential oil not only cleans but also leaves a fresh, citrus scent.

Tea Tree Essential Oil

Tea tree essential oil, derived from the leaves of the tea tree through steam distillation, is renowned for its potent antimicrobial properties. It is an excellent choice for cleaning surfaces, especially in areas like the bathroom, where sanitization is crucial.

Tea tree oil can effectively combat bacteria, viruses, and molds, making it a powerful tool in preventing the spread of germs. It can be used to clean bathroom counters, toilet seats, showers, and other bathroom surfaces. Here's a simple DIY bathroom cleaner using tea tree essential oil:

Tea Tree Bathroom Cleaner Recipe:

- 1 cup water
- 1/2 cup distilled white vinegar
- 15-20 drops of tea tree essential oil

Mix the ingredients in a spray bottle and shake well. Spray the mixture onto the surfaces, let it sit for a few minutes, then wipe clean with a cloth. The tea tree oil will leave your bathroom fresh and sanitized.

Peppermint Essential Oil

Peppermint essential oil, extracted through steam distillation from the peppermint plant, has a refreshing and invigorating aroma. It is known for its antimicrobial properties and is an excellent choice for cleaning floors and windows.

Peppermint oil not only cleans effectively but also leaves a pleasant and uplifting scent. Here's a simple DIY floor cleaner using peppermint essential oil:

Peppermint Floor Cleaner Recipe:

- 2 cups water
- 1/4 cup white vinegar
- 10-15 drops of peppermint essential oil

Mix the ingredients in a bucket and use the solution to mop your floors. The peppermint oil will not only clean the floors but also leave behind a fresh and minty aroma.

These are just a few examples of how essential oils can be effectively used for surface cleaning. The beauty of essential oils lies in their versatility; you can experiment and create various cleaning solutions based on your preferences and cleaning needs.

Essential Oils for Laundry

Laundry is a routine chore, and using essential oils in your laundry routine can enhance the cleaning process, leaving your clothes smelling fresh and clean. Certain essential oils possess antibacterial properties, making them excellent additions to your laundry detergents and fabric softeners.

Lavender Essential Oil

Lavender essential oil, extracted from lavender flowers through steam distillation, is renowned for its calming and soothing properties. It is a popular choice for adding a delightful scent to laundry while also possessing mild antibacterial properties.

Adding lavender essential oil to your laundry can leave your clothes smelling wonderful and feeling soft. Here's how you can do it:

Lavender Laundry Freshener Recipe:

- Add a few drops of lavender essential oil to a small piece of cloth or a dryer ball.
- Toss it into the dryer with your laundry during the drying cycle.

The heat from the dryer will release the aroma of lavender, leaving your clothes with a subtle, pleasant scent.

Eucalyptus Essential Oil

Eucalyptus essential oil, derived from the leaves of the eucalyptus tree through steam distillation, has a refreshing and invigorating scent. It is known for its antibacterial and antifungal properties, making it an excellent choice for laundry, particularly for items like towels and linens.

Eucalyptus Laundry Refresher Recipe:

- Add a few drops of eucalyptus essential oil to a damp washcloth.
- Toss it into the dryer with your towels and linens during the drying cycle.

The eucalyptus oil will not only impart a fresh scent but also help eliminate any bacteria or odors from the laundry.

Incorporating essential oils into your laundry routine is a simple and effective way to naturally enhance the cleaning and freshening of your clothes. You can experiment with different oils and combinations to find the scents that you prefer.

Essential Oils for Air Freshening

Maintaining a fresh and pleasant-smelling home is an integral part of creating a welcoming atmosphere. Unfortunately, many commercial air fresheners contain harmful chemicals. Essential oils provide a safe and natural alternative to keeping your home smelling delightful.

Lavender Essential Oil

Lavender essential oil, in addition to its use in laundry, is a versatile oil for air freshening. It possesses a calming and soothing scent, making it an ideal choice for creating a serene atmosphere in your home.

Lavender Air Freshener Recipe:

- Add a few drops of lavender essential oil to a diffuser.
- Allow the diffuser to disperse the aroma throughout the room.

Alternatively, you can create a homemade air spray using lavender essential oil:

Lavender Air Spray Recipe:

- 1 cup distilled water
- 10-15 drops of lavender essential oil

Combine the ingredients in a spray bottle and shake well before each use. Spray the mixture into the air to freshen up any room with the calming aroma of lavender.

Citrus Essential Oils

Citrus essential oils, including lemon, orange, grapefruit, and lime, are well-known for their uplifting and refreshing scents. They are excellent choices for combating odors and leaving a clean, citrusy fragrance in the air.

Citrus Air Freshener Recipe:

- Add a few drops of your preferred citrus essential oil(s) to a diffuser.
- Allow the diffuser to disperse the uplifting aroma throughout the room.

You can also create a simple DIY citrus air spray:

Citrus Air Spray Recipe:

- 1 cup distilled water
- 10-15 drops of your preferred citrus essential oil(s)

Mix the ingredients in a spray bottle and shake well. Use this spray to refresh the air in any room.

Incorporating essential oils for air freshening not only enhances the ambiance of your home but also provides therapeutic benefits, promoting a sense of well-being and relaxation.

Essential oils offer a natural, safe, and aromatic approach to cleaning and freshening your home. From their effectiveness in surface cleaning to their contribution to laundry and air freshening, essential oils are versatile tools that can transform your household cleaning routine.

Essential Oils for Home Care

Essential oils have been gaining popularity not only for their aromatic qualities but also for their versatile applications in home care. These potent extracts, derived from various plants, have been utilized for centuries to address a wide array of needs, from personal well-being to household maintenance.

Essential Oils in Personal Care

Essential oils have made a significant impact in the realm of personal care, owing to their natural properties and pleasant fragrances. As individuals become more conscious of the products they use on their bodies, essential oils have emerged as a key ingredient in a wide range of personal care products.

Lavender Essential Oil for Skincare

Lavender essential oil, obtained from the lavender plant, is a popular choice in skincare products due to its gentle nature and versatile benefits. Lavender oil is known for its calming and soothing effects on the skin, making it an ideal ingredient for various skincare applications.

Incorporating lavender essential oil into your skincare routine can help alleviate skin irritations, reduce redness, and promote a clear complexion. Its antimicrobial properties make it effective for treating acne, while its soothing qualities can relieve skin conditions such as eczema and psoriasis.

To create a simple lavender-infused skincare product, combine a few drops of lavender essential oil with a carrier oil, such as jojoba or coconut oil. This mixture can be used as a gentle facial moisturizer or a soothing massage oil.

Tea Tree Essential Oil for Acne Treatment

Tea tree essential oil, derived from the leaves of the tea tree, is renowned for its powerful antibacterial and antifungal properties. It has become a staple ingredient in many acne-fighting products due to its ability to combat acne-causing bacteria and reduce inflammation.

When applied topically, tea tree oil can help treat acne breakouts and promote clearer skin. However, it's important to use it in moderation and properly dilute it with carrier oil to avoid skin irritation.

To create a tea tree oil acne treatment, mix a few drops of tea tree essential oil with a carrier oil and apply it to the affected areas. Alternatively, you can add a drop or two of tea tree oil to your regular face cleanser for an added acne-fighting boost.

Peppermint Essential Oil for Hair Care

Peppermint essential oil, known for its refreshing and invigorating aroma, is also beneficial for hair care. It can help stimulate the scalp, improve blood circulation, and promote hair growth. Additionally, peppermint oil has a cooling effect, making it particularly soothing for an itchy or irritated scalp.

To incorporate peppermint essential oil into your hair care routine, add a few drops to your shampoo or conditioner. Gently massage it into your scalp to enjoy its stimulating and revitalizing effects.

Essential Oils for Pest Control

Pests are a common concern in households, and the use of chemical-laden pesticides raises environmental and health concerns. Essential oils offer a natural and effective solution for managing pests without the adverse effects associated with conventional pest control methods.

Citronella Essential Oil for Mosquito Repellent

Citronella essential oil is well-known for its ability to repel mosquitoes. It is a natural alternative to commercial mosquito repellents, which often contain harmful chemicals. Citronella oil emits a strong and pleasant aroma that deters mosquitoes and other flying insects.

To create a homemade mosquito repellent, mix citronella essential oil with a carrier oil, such as coconut oil, and apply it to exposed areas of your skin before heading outdoors. You can also use citronella oil in diffusers to deter mosquitoes from entering your living spaces.

Peppermint Essential Oil for Ant Control

Ants can be persistent invaders in homes, particularly during warmer months. Peppermint essential oil is an effective natural deterrent for ants due to its strong scent, which ants find displeasing and overwhelming.

To deter ants, prepare a peppermint oil spray by mixing a few drops of peppermint essential oil with water. Spray this mixture along windowsills, doorways, and other areas where ants may enter. Additionally, you can soak cotton balls in peppermint oil and place them in strategic locations to keep ants at bay.

Aromatherapy and Well-being

Aromatherapy, a practice that utilizes the therapeutic properties of essential oils through inhalation and topical application, plays a crucial role in promoting overall well-being and emotional balance.

Lavender Essential Oil for Relaxation and Sleep

Lavender essential oil is renowned for its calming and sedative properties, making it a popular choice for promoting relaxation and aiding sleep. The scent of lavender can help reduce stress, anxiety, and insomnia, allowing for a peaceful and restful night's sleep.

To enjoy the relaxing benefits of lavender essential oil, add a few drops to a diffuser before bedtime or place a drop on your pillow. You can also create a calming bath by adding a few drops of lavender oil to warm bathwater.

Eucalyptus Essential Oil for Respiratory Health

Eucalyptus essential oil is widely recognized for its benefits in supporting respiratory health. Its invigorating aroma can help clear congestion and promote easier breathing, making it an excellent choice during cold and flu seasons.

To experience the respiratory benefits of eucalyptus oil, add a few drops to a bowl of hot water and inhale the steam. Alternatively, use a diffuser to disperse the oil into the air, providing relief for congestion and respiratory discomfort.

CONCLUSION

In this final stretch of our aromatic journey through *The Essential Oils and Aromatherapy Bible*, we find ourselves at a crossroads of knowledge and wonder. Having traversed the intricate realms of essential oils and the art of aromatherapy, we stand on the verge of a newfound appreciation for nature's profound offerings.

Through the preceding chapters, we've delved deep into the world of essential oils, exploring their origins, extraction methods, and the diverse array of oils available. We've unveiled the therapeutic properties that these oils possess, empowering us to alleviate ailments, uplift moods, and enhance our overall well-being. The chapters have been a trove of wisdom, revealing the secrets of blending, application techniques, and safety precautions, ensuring that we utilize these potent gifts responsibly and effectively.

As we close this remarkable volume, we reflect upon the transformative journey we've undertaken. The *Essential Oils and Aromatherapy Bible* has been a beacon of enlightenment, illuminating the potential of harnessing nature's aromas for a harmonious and healthier life. Our expedition began with a simple notion: a curiosity about the scents that fill the air and their potential to influence our lives profoundly. Little did we know then that it would unfurl into an odyssey of knowledge, a voyage through the aromatic tapestry of existence.

From the aromatic gardens and distillation processes to the therapeutic wonders and the art of blending, we've seen the facets of essential oils and aromatherapy come alive. The ancient practices that have withstood the test of time now find a place of reverence in our modern lives. We've learned to embrace the holistic benefits that these natural essences offer, appreciating their ability to nurture our bodies, minds, and spirits.

This book has been a guide, a mentor, and a companion in this expedition. It has provided us with the tools and understanding needed to navigate the world of essential oils and aromatherapy confidently. Armed with this knowledge, we can curate blends that suit our unique needs, harnessing the power of aromas to boost our vitality, create a serene environment, and enhance our beauty. We've discovered that the possibilities are as vast as the fragrant gardens themselves.

The journey doesn't end here, though. Rather, it evolves into a lifelong exploration and integration of the principles and practices we've uncovered. We are now equipped to spread this wisdom, sharing the transformative power of essential oils with our loved ones, enriching their lives in turn.

As we bid farewell to this book, we carry forth the essence of its teachings. We carry the power of nature's aromas within us, a gentle reminder that the beauty and healing properties of the natural world are always within reach. With each inhalation, we embrace the therapeutic magic of essential oils, allowing it to permeate our being and elevate our existence.

INDEX

Made in United States
Troutdale, OR
05/06/2024

19675775R00117